Terry Priestman

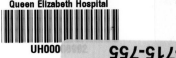

Cancer Chemotherapy in Clinical Practice

Second Edition

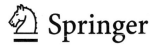 Springer

Terry Priestman, MD
FRCP, FRCR
New Cross Hospital
Wolverhampton
UK

ISBN 978-0-85729-726-6   ISBN 978-0-85729-727-3 (eBook)
ISBN 978-1-84628-989-7   ISBN 978-1-84628-991-0 (eBook)
DOI 10.1007/978-0-85729-727-3
Springer Dordrecht Heidelberg New York London

Library of Congress Control Number: 2012939623

A catalogue record for this book is available from the British Library

Printed on acid-free paper

Springer is part of Springer Science+Business Media (www.springer.com)

Preface

This book is intended as a basic overview of the drug treatment of cancer for junior doctors and specialist nurses who come into contact with people having chemotherapy as part of their day to day work. The aim is to provide a context to those treatments, explaining what the drugs are, how they work, some of their more likely side effects, how they are used in the treatment of the commoner cancers, and what therapeutic results might be expected.

The first use of the word chemotherapy is credited to Paul Ehrlich (1854–1915), who used it to describe the arsenical compounds he developed to treat syphilis. Nowadays when people talk about 'chemotherapy', as part of cancer treatment, they are usually referring to the use of cytotoxic drugs. Cytotoxics have dominated systemic cancer therapy for the last 50 years, and their use has resulted in enormous improvements in outcome. But they are only one component of the drug treatment of malignancy. Hormonal therapies are another major contributor to increased cure rates and survival times, and the last decade has seen an explosion of entirely new types of drugs for cancer treatment. The latter are mainly drugs specifically targeted against cancer cells (whereas cytotoxics affect both normal and malignant cells). These newer compounds have sometimes been popularly termed 'magic bullets', which again takes us back to Ehrlich, as this was another phrase he used to describe his treatments.

The aim of this text is to cover all these different elements of systemic therapy, giving an explanation of their various modes of action, their side effects, and their place in the everyday treatment of common cancers, with the hope of offering a simple overview of an increasingly complex, diverse, and incredibly exciting area of modern-day medicine.

While some cytotoxic and hormonal agents have been in common use for more than 50 years, many of the treatments described in this book have only appeared in the last 5 years, and others remain prospects for the future. The recent rapid expansion of therapeutic options for systemic cancer treatment, with drugs having a range of new lines of attack on the process of cancer growth, has meant that there is no universally agreed system for classifying these therapies. Because some of the newer agents only affect cancer cells and cause relatively little damage to normal tissue (in contrast to the established cytotoxic drugs) they have been called 'targeted' therapies. Another phrase that is used is 'biological therapies' or 'biological response modifiers'; some authorities restrict this to describing the cytokines, whilst others use it to embrace a far wider range of compounds, including all the monoclonal antibodies. As a result the current terminology can be confusing, and is still evolving. I have adopted the approach of trying to show how all these different options we now have for attacking cancer relate to the basic process of tumour growth and development.

Details of specific drug dose and treatment schedules are deliberately not given. This is partly because there is often considerable variation from hospital to hospital on the precise dosage and timing of treatment, even with 'standard' therapies, but also because the prescription of most of the drugs described in this book is restricted to experienced specialist clinicians and would not normally be the responsibility of more junior doctors. So whilst it is important for them to be aware of what the drugs are and why they are being used, it is not anticipated that the readers of this book would be involved in either the choice of treatment or its prescription. Throughout the text I have used the approved names (non-proprietary) names of the drugs. The UK proprietary (trade) names are given in Appendix A.

In the brief space of 4 years since the first edition of this book was written, there has been a plethora of new drugs either becoming available in routine clinical practice or entering clinical trials for people with cancer. This has increased the treatment options in many conditions although often with only a modest improvement in outcomes.

One of the most important concepts to have emerged during this time is that of personalised therapy. This is the hope that in the not too distant future it might be possible to use the biology of the individual patient's cancer to determine the treatment that should be given. For many years the only guide in this direction was the presence or absence of oestrogen receptors in breast cancers as an indicator of their hormonal sensitivity, this was followed in the 1990s by the discovery of the HER2 receptor over-expression as a marker for sensitivity to trastuzumab in the same condition. But in the last few years we have come to appreciate that newer drugs for common cancers like bowel and lung cancer are dependent on the presence or absence of specific gene mutations for their effectiveness and so can be targeted to specific subgroups of patients. The concept of gene array assay, the first clinical results of which have been reported in a number of recent papers, offers the hope that in a few years it will be possible to use the genetic profile of an individual's cancer to define a specific programme of therapy for them rather than rely on data based on large cohorts of patients.

This is largely for the future, but in the interim treatment choices still have to be made. In the past these were based on the clinical judgement of individual oncologists, but the last two decades have seen an increasing focus on evidence-based decision making. Initially this relied on the results of clinical trials, and then increasingly on meta-analyses of a series of studies and more recently on the guidelines produced by authoritative bodies.

The production of guidelines is of great potential benefit in unifying approaches to treatment and raising standards of care. But they do present at least two problems. Firstly, there is the increasing number of these documents. In the UK for example there are European guidelines, then national guidelines, regional guidelines (produced by each of the Cancer

Networks) and guidelines issued by various professional collaborations. Although these will have a broad consensus on the management of specific cancers they will often vary in their detail and will be different again from guidelines produced in the USA and elsewhere outside Europe. So the available guidelines are not entirely consistent. Secondly, they can never be completely up to date: they rely on evidence for their validity and meta-analyses of clinical trials are the strongest form of that evidence. But clinical trials take years to design, recruit, mature and be published, and by the time a sufficient number are available for meta-analysis new drugs might be available which may or may not improve the chances of a benefit for the patient to be treated. So at the end of the day clinical judgement still is not dead, it has to be continuously used to weigh up the available evidence in order to make individual treatment decisions.

Another factor that is increasingly overshadowing oncological decision making is money. In the past clinicians have usually been free to make choices based on what they believe to be best for their patient. But the increasing cost of cancer drugs has challenged this situation. Although there have been a few major breakthroughs, many of the new drugs offer the hope of only a few extra weeks of life at a cost of thousands, if not tens of thousands of dollars or pounds. At a time of global economic downturn the value of these treatments has been subject to scrutiny. For some years in England and Wales only those drugs approved by NICE (the National Institute for Clinical Excellence) on the basis not only of their efficacy but also cost-effectiveness have been available on prescription on the National Health Service, with the result that many anti-cancer drugs available in other countries have not been routinely available to NHS patients (this situation partly changed in 2010 with the introduction of the government's Cancer Drugs Fund to help provide drugs not approved by NICE, but the implementation of that programme across the country has been patchy leading to a new form of postcode lottery in cancer treatment). With continuing global economic problems and financial constraints, and the continuing escalation of drug costs, an increasing number of experts and professional organisations in the USA the UK and across the world have voiced concerns about the apparently limitless increase in the financial burden of cancer care; this issue is likely to impact on clinical practice and therapeutic choice in the years to come.

To be aware of all the current data from clinical trials, the recommendations of guidelines and the economic constraints on prescribing in addition to an understanding of the fundamental principles of oncology and to use this knowledge to formulate a treatment plan in the best interest of the individual patient is the skill demanded of the modern-day oncologist. It is not the role of this book to provide the information to inform their decisions; that would require at the very least a major textbook of great length. This book is intended for those members of the team who are not the specialist decision makers: the junior doctors, nurses, students and other health professionals who want to have some understanding of the background information and clinical context that shapes the treatment plans they are asked to help implement on a day-to-day basis; it is an attempt at a simple, brief, introduction to a subject of huge and ever increasing complexity.

March 2012   Terry Priestman

Contents

Chapter 1
The Theoretical Basis
of Cancer Chemotherapy

Historical Introduction

The first drugs to treat cancer effectively were the hormonal
and cytotoxic agents which appeared in the early 1940s.

In 1896 the Glasgow surgeon, George Beatson, reported
the remission of an advanced breast cancer in a young woman,
following removal of her ovaries. In a parallel discovery, just
over 40 years later, Charles Huggins, working in Chicago,
showed that prostate cancer would regress following castration.
Shortly before this, in 1938, Charles Dodds, in London, had
produced a synthetic form of the female hormone oestrogen:
stilboestrol. In 1941 Huggins showed that, like castration, stilboestrol could cause prostate cancer to regress, and in 1944
Alexander Haddow reported the successful use of the drug to
treat women with metastatic breast cancer.

At the same time other pioneers were building on the First
World War observation that the poison gas, sulphur mustard,
caused shrinkage of lymphoid tissue, and a fall in the white
blood cell count, as well as many other effects. In 1942
Goodman and Gilman, working at Yale, used nitrogen mustard, a derivative of sulphur mustard, to treat a man with
advanced lymphoma: his cancer briefly regressed.

Stilboestrol and nitrogen mustard opened the flood gates,
and over the last 60 years more than a 100 hormonal and
cytotoxic agents have been developed for cancer treatment.

These early breakthroughs were based on empirical observations; why the treatments worked was a mystery. Relatively

T. Priestman, *Cancer Chemotherapy in Clinical Practice*,
DOI 10.1007/978-0-85729-727-3_1,
© Springer-Verlag London 2012

quickly it was realised that nitrogen mustard, and the numerous other cytotoxic agents that followed in its wake, acted by directly interfering with the process of cell division; inhibiting mitosis in one way or another. But it was not until the 1958 that Elwood Jensen discovered oestrogen receptors (ER), providing a basis for understanding the hormonal sensitivity of some cancers.

We now know that about two out of three breast cancers are made up of cells carrying ER (ER+ cancers). Those ER bind circulating oestrogen, and in so doing are stimulated to promote cell division: the cancer is hormone dependant for its growth. In the same way, it has been discovered that most prostate cancers carry receptors for the male hormone, androgen, and this drives their growth.

The receptor story gives us an insight into more recent developments in the drug treatment of cancer. In 1977 the epidermal growth factor receptor (EGFR) was identified, the first of a number of tyrosine kinase receptors which have been found in many different types of cancer. This has led to the development of at least three lines of therapeutic attack. The first of these has focused on reducing the levels of circulating growth factors which stimulate these receptors. The second approach has been to explore ways of blocking or inhibiting receptors, so they cannot be stimulated. The third approach has looked at the next stage in the pathway of cell growth: when a receptor is stimulated it then sends a message to the cell nucleus, telling it to make the cell divide. This is known as signal transduction. Much research in recent years has been focused on identifying the chemical messengers that link the receptor to the nucleus, carrying the signals for cell division, and now the first drugs are appearing that can disrupt these chemicals, and break the chain of communication between the receptor and the nucleus.

This brief history identifies the key milestones in the development of cancer chemotherapy. It also indicates how the discovery of new systemic treatments for cancer has been paralleled by an increasing understanding of tumour biology. The latter now gives us a clear picture of the natural history of cancers, from their origin, at a molecular level, in genetic mutations, to the impact those changes have on the mechanisms controlling cell growth, and a knowledge of subsequent tumour kinetics, which leads to the appearance of clinically

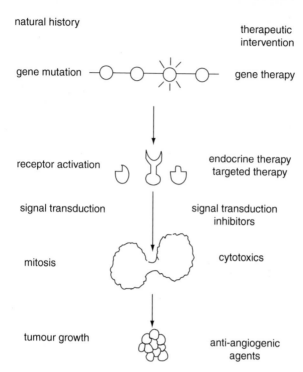

natural history

therapeutic
intervention

gene mutation   gene therapy

receptor activation   endocrine therapy
targeted therapy

signal transduction   signal transduction
inhibitors

mitosis   cytotoxics

tumour growth   anti-angiogenic
agents

FIGURE 1.1 The natural history of cancer and the place of different chemotherapeutic interventions

obvious, potentially lethal, malignancies. To fill in more detail about the types of anti-cancer drugs that are used now, and might be used in the future, and to explain how they work the approach we will adopt is to look at the natural history of cancer, and relate the different types of systemic therapy to the various stages of cancer development (see Fig. 1.1).

Suggestions for Further Reading

Chabner BA, Roberts TG. Chemotherapy and the war on cancer. Nat Rev Cancer. 2005;5:65–72.

Hirsch J. An anniversary for cancer chemotherapy. JAMA. 2006;296:1518–20.

Thomas A. Joe Burchenal and the birth of combination chemotherapy. Br J Haematol. 2006;133:493–503.

In the Beginning: Genes

Cancers begin as the result of an abnormality in the genes of one or more cells in the body. That abnormality may either be inherited, the faulty gene being passed from one generation to the next, or acquired, a normal gene being damaged or mutating for some reason.

Three types of genes have been identified which have a role in cancer formation: oncogenes, tumour suppressor genes and caretaker genes. When an oncogene mutates it switches on the process of uncontrolled cell division which leads to a cancer. Tumour suppressor genes, as their name implies, normally regulate the process of cell replication, keeping it under control, when they mutate that control is lost, the brakes are off, and once again uncontrolled cell division occurs. Caretaker genes are responsible for maintaining the integrity of DNA, when they mutate DNA damage can accumulate without being repaired and ultimately lead to cancer development.

The first gene to be shown to be directly related to cancer development was the RB-1, retinoblastoma, gene, abnormalities of which lead to the childhood cancer of the same name, which affects the retina. This is a rare tumour, but among the more common cancers we now know that about 1 in 20 breast cancers result from mutations in either the BRCA1 or BRCA2 gene, and about 1 in 20 bowel cancers result from changes in the FPC (familial polyposis coli) gene, or the HNPCC (hereditary non-polyposis coli) gene. The retinoblastoma, and FPC genes are tumour suppressor genes and the BRCA1, BRCA2 and HNPCC genes are caretaker genes. ('HNPCC gene' is actually a collective term for a group of genes, known as mismatch repair, or mmr genes, including MSH1, MSH2 and MSH6, mutations in any of which may lead to HNPCC).

All the genes mentioned so far are inherited but two very important genes which are commonly mutated in sporadic cancers (Table 1.1) are the P53 and KRAS. The P53 is a tumour suppressor gene and KRAS is an oncogene.

TABLE 1.1 Percentage of sporadic cancers with P53 or KRAS mutations

	P53 (%)	KRAS (%)
Lung	70	20
Colon	60	40
Prostate	30	
Ovary	60	17
Breast	20	
Bladder	60	
Pancreas		70

TABLE 1.2 Some ways in which anti-cancer gene therapy might be used

Replacing faulty genes: inserting new normal genes into the cells to replace the abnormal cancerous genes

Boosting immunity: altering the cancer genes to make their cells more vulnerable to the body's immune system

Increasing sensitivity to treatment: altering the cancer genes to make their cells either more vulnerable to other treatments, or to stop them developing resistance to those treatments

Reducing the sensitivity of normal cells to treatment: selectively targeting normal genes to make their cells more resistant to the effects of treatment, so that higher doses of drugs or radiation may be given

Suicide genes: introducing genes into cancer cells which are designed to destroy the abnormal oncogenes or tumour suppressor genes

Anti-angiogenesis genes: introducing genes into cancer cells that will stop them from developing the new blood vessels essential for the support of tumour growth

At the present time an ever increasing number of genes are being discovered, mutations of which may lead to cancer. The identification of these genetic abnormalities opens the way for a whole new approach to cancer treatment: gene therapy. There are a number of ways in which this could be used (Table 1.2) but at the moment exploiting these is very much at the research stage, either in the laboratory or the most preliminary of clinical trials. It will be some years until we know whether targeting genes will produce therapeutic results, but already progress is being made in a different direction: using the knowledge of gene mutations to select specific treatments (see page 36).

Suggestions for Further Reading

Croce CM. Oncogenes and cancer. N Engl J Med. 2008;358:502–12.
Hainaut P, Wiman KG. 30 years and a long way into p53 research. Lancet Oncol. 2009;10:913–19.
Linardou H, Briasoulis E, Dahabreh IJ, et al. All about KRAS for clinical oncology practice. Cancer Treat Rev. 2010;37:221–33.

Growth Factors and Receptors

We all begin our lives as a single fertilized cell. That cell then divides to form two cells, those two cells divide to make four, and this process of cell division continues throughout pregnancy, and on through infancy, childhood and adolescence, to produce the countless billions of cells that make up our adult selves. The process of cell growth continues in adulthood, because cells are constantly wearing out and dying off and need to be replaced. Throughout our lives, this process of cell division is very precisely controlled so that we make exactly the right number of new cells that our bodies need – no more, no less. A cancer develops when the cells in a particular organ escape from these controls and begin to reproduce and grow in a haphazard way, producing more cells than they should.

Key components of the control process for cell division are growth factors and receptors. Growth factors are chemicals which circulate in the blood stream and bind to specific receptor sites on the cell surface or in the cellular cytoplasm. The resulting interaction between the growth factor and the receptor then triggers the next step in stimulating cell division.

Faulty genes can affect the growth factor-receptor system in a number of ways. For example they can cause an overproduction, or over-expression, of growth factor receptors. This effectively makes the cell far more sensitive to natural growth factors, which stimulate them to multiply excessively. Alternatively they may lead receptors to be active even when they are not being stimulated by growth factors.

At the present time the two families of receptors that are of major importance in oncology are steroid receptors and the tyrosine kinase receptors.

Steroid Receptors and Endocrine Therapy

The two main steroid receptors related to cancer growth are oestrogen and androgen receptors. About two out of three breast cancers are made up of cells carrying an abnormally high level of oestrogen receptors, they are ER+, similarly more than nine out of ten prostate cancers have an over expression of androgen receptors. These receptor positive cancers rely on circulating hormone to stimulate their growth. Oestrogen or androgen interact with the receptors to produce chemical signals which trigger the process of mitosis (see Fig. 1.2).

Oestrogen and androgen could be thought of as the first cancer growth factors to be recognized, although they are not normally classified in that way.

Therapeutically this hormonally-driven cancer growth can be inhibited in two ways: either by reducing the level of circulating hormone, or by blocking the receptor so that the hormonal growth factor cannot reach it. In premenopausal women circulating oestrogen levels may be reduced either by inhibition of sex hormone production by the pituitary gland (using gonaderilin analogues) or by ablation of the ovaries, by surgery or radiotherapy. The gonaderilin analogues (also known as LHRH, luteinising hormone-releasing hormone, analogues) initially stimulate pituitary receptors, leading to a transient increase in luteinising hormone, and hence sex hormone, levels, before down-regulating the receptors, rendering them

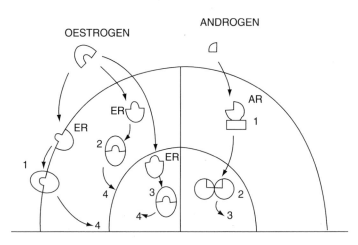

FIGURE 1.2 Oestrogen and androgen receptor signalling pathways. Circulating oestrogen binds to oestrogen receptors (*ER*) in the cell membrane, in the cytoplasm or in the nucleus to form membrane (*1*), mitochondrial (*2*) or nuclear (*3*) oestrogen-receptor complexes, which then trigger the release of signalling proteins (*4*) to stimulate DNA synthesis and cell division. Androgen receptors (*AR*) are in the cytoplasm, bound to a protein which inactivates them (*1*). Androgen releases the receptor from the protein and it moves to the cell nucleus where receptors form pairs (dimerize) (*2*) and bind to androgen-response elements which trigger the release of signalling proteins to stimulate DNA synthesis and cell division (*3*)

insensitive. Although ovarian production of oestrogen ceases with the menopause the hormone is still produced elsewhere in the body, especially in the fatty tissues, where androgen, secreted by the adrenal gland is converted into oestrogen (see Fig. 1.3). This synthesis involves the aromatase enzymes, and their inhibition leads to a fall in oestrogen levels. So the aromatase inhibitors reduce oestrogen levels in older women. By contrast tamoxifen acts at all ages by blocking the oestrogen receptor itself. This statement is a slight oversimplification of tamoxifen's action, as although it does competitively block ER on cancer cells it actually has a stimulatory effect on other ER, for example those in the endometrium, lining the womb. This more complex relationship with ER is reflected in an

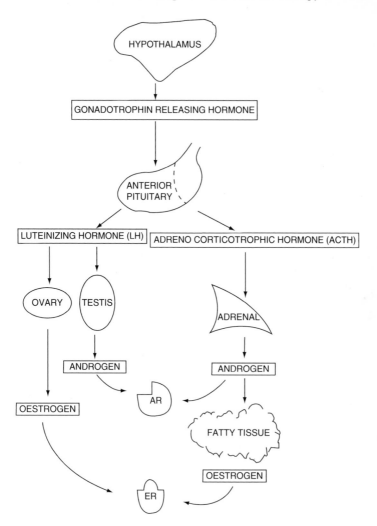

FIGURE 1.3 Hormonal pathways for oestrogen and androgen production. Before the menopause luteinising hormone (*LH*) stimulates production of androgens in the ovary which are converted to oestrogen by the aromatase enzyme pathway. After the menopause oestrogen production continues, at a much reduced level, by conversion of androgen secreted by the adrenals carried out by aromatase enzymes mainly in the fatty tissues

TABLE 1.3 Hormonal agents

Mode of action	Breast cancer	Prostate cancer
Pituitary inhibitors	Goserilin	Goserilin
		Leuprorelin
		Degarelix
Inhibitors of hormone synthesis		Abiraterone
Competitive receptor inhibitors	Tamoxifen	Bicalutamide
	Toremifene	Cyproterone
		Flutamide
Receptor downregulation	Fulvestrant	
Aromatase inhibition	Anastrazole	
	Exemestane	
	Letrozole	
Multiple modes of action	Progestogens	Diethyl-stilboestrol
	Megestrol acetate	
	Medroxyprogesterone acetate	

alternative description of tamoxifen as a selective estrogen receptor modulator (SERM).

Another group of hormones which have activity in breast cancer are the progestogens, synthetic forms of the female hormone progesterone (see Table 1.3). Although some breast cancer cells do carry specific progestogen receptors (PgR+ cancers) the interaction of the drugs with these is probably of secondary importance in their anti-tumour effect as they also have a number of other properties including reducing ovarian and adrenal androgen production, reducing the expression of ER, and, possibly, a direct cytotoxic action on breast cancer cells.

In prostate cancer gonaderilin analogues or surgical castration are established methods of reducing circulating androgen levels. They have recently been joined by the oral agent abiraterone which works by inhibiting the enzyme

17α-hydroxylase/C17.20 lyase (CYP17A1) which is instrumental in androgen synthesis and thereby lowers circulating testosterone levels. Then there are the anti-androgenic agents which mimic the action of tamoxifen in competing for receptors on the cancer cell. These latter drugs are classified as either steroidal (cyproterone acetate) or non-steroidal (flutamide, bicalutamide). Because of its steroidal properties cyproterone also causes some pituitary inhibition of hormone production as well as the competitive inhibition of androgen receptors. A consequence of these slightly differing modes of action is that the non-steroidal anti-androgens do not lower circulating androgen levels whilst cyproterone does, and this affects the side-effect profile of the drugs (see page 67). In the early days of systemic therapy for prostate cancer stilboestrol was the drug of choice. This acts in a number of ways, including reduction of LHRH secretion, inactivation of circulating androgen and direct suppression of androgen production by the testes, it has also been suggested that it may be directly cytotoxic to tumour cells in the prostate. Although the drug fell out of favour for many years because of a high level of thromboembolic complications it has now regained a place as an effective third or fourth line treatment in metastatic prostate cancer.

Another family of hormone receptors is the glucocorticoid receptors. These are found in the cytoplasm of lymphocytes and are the target of the corticosteroids prednisone, prednisolone and dexamethasone. When the corticosteroid binds to the receptors the steroid-receptor complex moves to the cell nucleus and activates programmed cell death (apoptosis). In this way giving steroids reduces the number of lymphocytes, and this forms the basis for their use in a number of haematological cancers.

Suggestions for Further Reading

Chen Y, Clegg NJ, Scher HI. Anti-androgen and androgen depleting therapies. Lancet Oncol. 2009;10:981–92.

Chmelar R, Buchanan G, Need EF, et al. Androgen receptor coregulators and their involvement in the development and progression of prostate cancer. Int J Cancer. 2007;120:719–33.

Debes JD, Tindall DJ. Mechanisms of androgen-refractory prostate cancer. N Engl J Med. 2004;351:1488–90.
Yager JD, Davidson NE. Estrogen carcinogenesis in breast cancer. N Engl J Med. 2006;354:270–82.

Tyrosine Kinase Genes

The human genome contains more than 100 tyrosine kinase (TK) genes. These genes produce tyrosine kinases which are a family of enzymes involved in the regulation of cell division (mitosis), programmed cell death (apoptosis), and a number of other cellular functions. There are a number of different families of TK genes, and three of these in particular play a crucial part in the growth of certain cancers, these are the epidermal growth factor receptors (EGFR), vascular endothelial growth factor receptors (VEGFR), and non-receptor tyrosine kinases. The EGF and VEGF receptors have similar structure, as shown in Fig. 1.4.

EGFR

EGFRs are a family of receptors made up of EGFR, HER2, HER3 and HER4. EGFRs are found in normal epithelial cells, and are stimulated by a number of different growth factors the two most important of which are epidermal growth factor (EGF) and transforming growth factor α (TGF-α). Incidentally, the compounds which bind to, and stimulate, these receptors are often referred to as ligands.

EGFRs are made up of three parts, or domains: an extracellular domain, which binds the circulating growth factors, a transmembrane domain, which crosses the cell membrane, and an intracellular (tyrosine kinase) domain. Stimulation causes the receptors to form into pairs (this is called, dimerization). Dimerization leads to a change in the structure of the receptors which then triggers the intracellular domain to activate a biochemical pathway in which the tyrosine kinase enzymes are the key component (see Fig. 1.5).

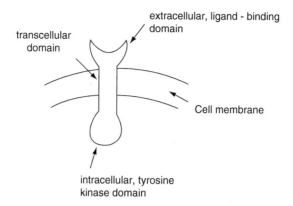

FIGURE 1.4 The basic structure of a tyrosine kinase (*TK*) receptor. The extracellular domain is the target for monoclonal antibodies like cetuximab, bevacizumab or trastuzumab. The intracellular domain is the target for small molecule TK inhibitors like erlotinib, gefitinib and lapatinib

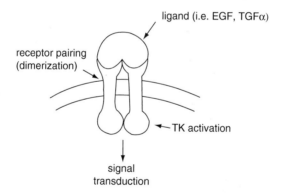

FIGURE 1.5 Activation of EGFR family receptors. Dimerization may be between two of the same receptors, i.e. EGFR and EGFR (homodimerization), or two different receptors, i.e. EGFR and HER2 (heterodimerization). HER2 has no known ligands, and is activated by heterodimerization, although if HER2 is heavily over-expressed it can form homodimers which can activate the TK signalling pathway without ligand binding (autoactivation). The intracellular domain of HER3 has no TK component, but HER3 can activate signal transduction by forming heterodimers with other EGFRs

TABLE 1.4 The epidermal growth factor receptor family

Receptor	Alternative names	Over-expressed in these cancers
EGFR	HER1[a]	Head and neck (90%)
	erbB1[b]	Kidney, clear cell (70%)
	ErbB1	Lung, non-small cell (60%)
		Breast, ovary, colorectal (50%)
		Pancreas, bladder, prostate (40%)
HER2	erbB2	Breast (20%)
	ErbB2	Endometrial (15%)
	HER2/neu	Ovary
	c-erbB-2	Cervical (15%)
HER3	erbB3	Breast, colon, stomach, prostate, soft tissue sarcoma
	ErbB3	
HER4	erbB4	Breast, prostate, medulloblastoma
	ErbB4	

[a]HER: an abbreviation of human epidermal growth factor
[b]erbB: this has its origin in the fact that EGFR was discovered through work on oncogenes present in the avian erythroblastosis gene (v-erbB)

Both EGFR and HER2 have been linked to a number of cancers (Table 1.4). Genetic mutations can affect these receptors in a number of ways, the most important of which is over expression, producing an excess of the receptors in the cell, which makes that cell abnormally sensitive to circulating growth factors.

Looking for drugs that will inhibit the EGFR system is one of the most active areas of research in oncology at present. So far two types of agent have been developed: monoclonal antibodies which bind to and block the extracellular receptor domain, and small-molecule EGFR tyrosine kinase inhibitors (TKIs), which suppress the activation of the intracellular domain (Table 1.5).

TABLE 1.5 EGFR family inhibitors

Drug	Type	Receptor/domain targeted	Formulation
Cetuximab	moab[a]	EGFR/extracellular	iv
Trastuzumab	moab	HER2/extracellular	iv
Panitumumab	moab	EGFR/extracellular	iv
Pertuzumab	moab	HER2/extracellular	iv
Gefitinib	smtki[b]	EGFR/intracellular	Oral
Erlotinib	smtki	EGFR/intracellular	Oral
Lapatinib	smtki	EGFR & HER2/ intracellular	Oral

[a]Monoclonal antibody
[b]Small molecule tyrosine kinase inhibitor

A further development in recent years has been the discovery that some of the drugs inhibiting EGFR receptors (but not, so far, HER2 receptors) require the presence or absence of specific gene mutations in order to be effective. For example in people with non-small cell lung cancer only those who have specific EGFR mutations are likely to respond to the drugs erlotinib and gefitinib, whereas in people with colorectal cancer those who have a KRAS mutation are unlikely to respond to cetuximab or panitumumab whereas those who do not have this mutation may well benefit from the drugs.

VEGFR and Related Receptors

Once a cancer begins to grow then in order to survive it needs to develop its own blood supply. This involves creating new blood vessels, a process known as angiogenesis. The cells which form the capillaries are the endothelial cells. More than a dozen different chemicals have been identified that can be formed by cancers to stimulate angiogenesis. Three of the most important of these are vascular endothelial growth factor (VEGF), basic fibroblast growth factor (βFGF), and platelet-derived growth factor (PDGF). VEGF binds to two different receptors, VEGF

The angiogenic pathway

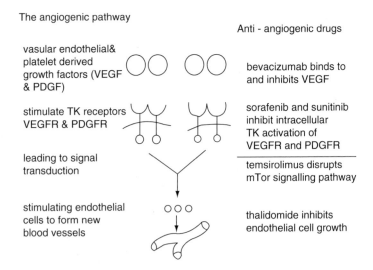

Anti - angiogenic drugs

vasular endothelial&
platelet derived
growth factors (VEGF
& PDGF)

bevacizumab binds to
and inhibits VEGF

stimulate TK receptors
VEGFR & PDGFR

sorafenib and sunitinib
inhibit intracellular
TK activation of
VEGFR and PDGFR

leading to signal
transduction

temsirolimus disrupts
mTor signalling pathway

stimulating endothelial
cells to form new
blood vessels

thalidomide inhibits
endothelial cell growth

FIGURE 1.6 The inhibition of tumour angiogenesis. Note: although not its main mode of action, imatinib is also an inhibitor of PDGFR

receptor type 1 and 2 (VEGFR-1, and VEGFR-2), and βFGF and PDGF both have their own receptors.

VEGF, βFGF and PDGF activation of their receptors stimulates tyrosine kinase activity which, among other things, releases enzymes called matrix metalloproteinases (MMPs) which breakdown the extracellular matrix: the supportive material that holds the cells together. This allows the endothelial cells to spread and multiply, thereby forming the new blood vessels.

Looking for agents that will suppress tumour angionesis is another current major research area, and once again monoclonal antibodies which block the receptors, have been developed as well as small-molecule tyrosine kinase inhibitors. As well as these agents that target the endothelial growth factor-receptor system other compounds are available, or in development which attack other aspects of the tumour vascularity. Collectively these drugs are known as anti-angiogenic agents, and they are summarized in Fig. 1.6. Sorafenib, sunitinib and pazopanib are of particular note as along with imatinib (which has a minor anti-angiogenic effect) they are multi-targeted

TABLE 1.6 Targeted therapies: multi-targeted drugs

Drug	Targets	Therapeutic indications
Imatinib	BCR-ABL	Chronic myeloid leukaemia
Nilotinib	KIT	Gastrointestinal stromal tumours (GIST)
Dasatinib	PDGFR	
Sorafenib	VEGFR	Renal cell cancer
	PDGFR	GIST
	KIT	
	MAPK/Ras	
Sunitinib	VEGFR	Renal cell cancer
	PDGFR	Hepatocellular cancer
	KIT	
	RET[a]	
Pazopanib	VEGFR	Renal cell cancer
	PDGFR	Ovarian cancer[b]
	KIT	Soft tissue sarcoma[b]

[a]A receptor linked to some neuroendocrine tumours
[b]Currently under investigation, value to be established

drugs, inhibiting a number of different components of the tyrosine kinase system (Table 1.6).

One particularly interesting member of this group is thalidomide, which achieved notoriety in the 1960s when its use in the treatment of morning sickness during pregnancy resulted in the birth defect phocomelia (failure of development of the long bones). It is now recognized that this toxicity was in part due to its antiangiogenic activity in the developing embryo. Thalidomide inhibits the transcription of angiogenic genes and thus prevents the formation of chemicals stimulating the process of new blood vessel formation. Thalidomide has proved an effective drug in the treatment of multiple myeloma but, for reasons that are not clear, has yet to show significant activity in other cancers. Apart from its teratogenic potential thalidomide does have other side effects, including peripheral neuropathy, drowsiness and constipation. A related drug, lenalidomide, has been developed which appears to have similar anti-angiogenic properties to thalidomide, and has shown activity in multiple myeloma and chronic lympho-cytic leukaemia.

Non-receptor Tyrosine Kinases

Unlike the EGF and VEGF receptors these tyrosine kinases exist in the cytoplasm, not on the surface of the cell, and have no receptor sites. Therefore they are not activated by the bind-ing of a growth factor, or ligand, but as a result of some cellular abnormality which leads to autostimulation, producing growth signalling proteins in the absence of any external stimulus. This mechanism has been most clearly demonstrated in a number of haematological cancers, where it occurs as a result of chro-mosomal translocations. The best studied of these is in chronic myeloid leukaemia, where 95% of patients have a transloca-tion between chromosomes 9 and 22, producing what is known as the Philadelphia chromosome. This translocation produces a fusion gene, BCR-ABL, the ABL gene then stimulates a specific non-receptor tyrosine kinase pathway which causes the leukaemic change. This process can be disrupted by a group of drugs which inhibit ABL thereby blocking the tyrosine kinase signalling pathway. The first of these drugs to come into clinical practice was imatinib and this has latterly been joined by niltonib and dasatinib. These agents often achieve a complete molecular response in chronic myeloid leukaemia with disappearance of the BCR-ABL gene.

Suggestions for Further Reading

Eichholz A, Merchant S, Gaya RM. Anti-angiogenesis therapies: their potential in cancer management. Onco Targets Ther. 2010;3:69–82.

Giardello F, Tortora G. EGFR antagonists in cancer treatment. N Engl J Med. 2008;358:1160–74.

Jones KL, Buzdar AV. Evolving novel antiHER2 strategies. Lancet Oncol. 2009;10:1179–87.

Kerbel RS. Molecular origins of cancer: tumor angiogenesis. N Engl J Med. 2008;358:2039–49.

Marshall J. Clinical implications of the mechanism of epidermal growth factor receptor inhibitors. Cancer. 2006;107:1207–18.

Mendelsohn J, Baselga J. Epidermal growth factor receptor targeting in cancer. Semin Oncol. 2006;33:369–85.

Rosa DD, Ismael G, Dal Lago L, Awada A. Molecular-targeted therapies: lessons from years of clinical development. Cancer Treat Rev. 2008;34:61–80.

Cytokines

Another group of compounds that could be considered as growth factors are the cytokines. Cytokines are an extensive family of naturally occurring proteins which play a part in regulating various aspects of the immune system, as well as a number of other physiological functions. Two cytokines have emerged as agents for anti-cancer therapy: interferon and interleukin. There is still controversy over the exact way in which these compounds affect cancer cells: some experts argue for a direct effect, whilst others suggest that they work by stimulating the immune system to attack the cancer. These uncertainties are reflected in the confusing terminology for these agents which have been referred to variously as biological response modifiers, biological therapies, immunomodulators or, simply, immunotherapy.

Monoclonal Antibodies Targeting Lymphocytes

Another group of biological therapies are monoclonal antibodies designed to target proteins on normal and malignant lymphocytes. Three compounds currently licensed in the UK are rituximab, alemtuzumab and ipilimumab. Rituximab and alemtuzumab target the CD20 and CD52 proteins respectively. These proteins are found on the surface of normal and malignant B lymphocytes, but are not present on normal stem cells, so that normal cells are readily replaced, with a minimum of toxicity. The monoclonal antibodies bind to the proteins, and this binding then acts as a signal to normal immune mechanisms to destroy the cells. Rituximab and alemtuzumab have a role in a number of haematological cancers. Ipilumumab binds to the protein CTLA-4 on cytotoxic T-lymphocytes. This binding stimulates the immune system to attack cancer cells. Ipilumumab has shown activity in malignant melanoma and prostate cancer.

Signal Transduction

Once a receptor has been stimulated it stimulates cell growth by sending a message to the cell nucleus which will lead to either mitosis, or inhibition of apoptosis. For steroid receptors there are a number of pathways but the classical interaction is a direct one, with hormones binding to receptors located in the cell nucleus. The EGFR and VEGFR families of receptors, located on the cell membrane, have to produce chemical messengers to travel to the nucleus to relay their stimulus. This process is called signal transduction. Once again multiple tyrosine kinase pathways play a key part in this process, and as these become identified so drugs can be developed to target them. Three signaling cascades have been identified as particularly important in cancer development, they are:

- mitogen-activated protein kinase (MAPK/Ras)
- phosphatidyl inositol-3-kinase (PI3K/AKT)
- protein kinase C (PKC)

Many drugs are under development as potential inhibitors of these pathways. Those which have already entered clinical practice include temsirolimus, and everolimus. These both inhibit the protein mTOR, which is a key component in the PI3K/AKT pathway. Sorafenib, which has already been mentioned as an anti-angiogenic drug, also inhibits Raf kinase, which is a key enzyme in the MAPK/ras signal transduction cascade. Another group of drugs which are being explored are the farnesyl transferase inhibitors. Farnesyl transferase is another key enzyme in the MAPK/Ras pathway. Tipifarnib and lonafarnib were drugs which were shown to inhibit farnesyl transferase and gave promising results in laboratory studies but have failed to show any significant benefit in clinical trials.

Suggestions for Further Reading

Le Tourneau C, Faivre S, Raymond E. New developments in multi-targeted therapy for patients with solid tumours. Cancer Treat Rev. 2008;34:37–48.

Schreck R, Rapp VR. Raf kinases: oncogenesis and drug discovery. Int J Cancer. 2006;119:2261–71.

Proteasome Inhibition

Proteasomes are enzyme complexes which are present in all cells. They degrade proteins that control a number of cellular activities, including the regulation of cell division. Inhibition of the proteasome interferes with the chemical signals which stimulate cell growth and replication. Cancer cells appear to be more sensitive to disturbance of proteasome function than normal cells. The first proteasome inhibitor to have been approved is bortezomib (Velcade), which has been shown to be of value in the treatment of multiple myeloma. Other proteasome inhibitors are in development and the proteasome is likely to be an increasingly important target for new cancer drugs.

Suggestion for Further Reading

Rajkumar SV, Richardson PG, Hideshima T, Anderson KC. Proteasome inhibition as a novel therapeutic target in human cancer. J Clin Oncol. 2005;23:630–9.

Mitosis: Cytotoxic Drugs

We now reach the stage in the carcinogenic pathway where the cell is stimulated to multiply in an uncontrolled fashion. The mechanism for that multiplication is the fundamental process of mitosis, with the duplication of the nuclear genetic material on the chromosomes and the subsequent formation of two new daughter cells from the one original. This is the point at which the classical cytotoxic chemotherapy drugs, the compounds which have evolved from the discovery of nitrogen mustard, take effect.

Cytotoxic drugs all act in one way or another to disrupt the process of mitosis. They do this in a variety of ways, and their mode of action forms a basis for their classification (Table 1.7).

Because cytotoxic drugs are still the major component of systemic anticancer therapy it is appropriate to describe here the mode of action of the main groups of drugs in a little more detail.

Alkylating Agents

Nitrogen mustard, the first cytotoxic drug to be identified in the 1940s (see page 1) is an alkylating agent. Within 20 years of its first application more than 3,000 other alkylating agents had been isolated for evaluation in cancer treatment. Of these 3,000 only a handful are in general use today.

An alkyl group is the chemical structure that results when an aliphatic or aromatic hydrocarbon loses one of its hydrogen atoms. The simplest of all alkyl groups has the formula CH_2. An alkylating agent is a compound that contains an alkyl group and is able to use that group to combine with other compounds by covalent bonds. At its simplest the general formula for an alkylating reaction, or alkylation is:

$$R - CH_2 - X + Y = R - CH_2 - Y + X$$

The principal action of cytotoxic alkylating agents is to attack the nitrogen atom at the N-7 position on the purine base guanine, in DNA and RNA. Most of the drugs possess

TABLE 1.7 A classification of cytotoxic drugs in common use

Alkylating agents

Bendamustine	Melphalan
Busulfan	Mitomycin[a]
Carmustine	Nitrogen mustard
Chlorambucil	Procarbazine
Cyclophosphamide	Temozolamide
Dacarbazine	Trabectedin
Ifosfamide	Treosulfan
Lomustine	

Platinum analogues

Carboplatin	Oxaliplatin
Cisplatin	

Antimetabolites

Capecitabine	Mercaptopurine
Cladribine	Methotrexate
Cytaribine	Pemetrexed
Fludarabine	Raltitrexed
Fluorouracil	Thioguanine
Gemcitabine	
Hydroxyurea	

Topoisomerase I inhibitors

Irinotecan	Topotecan

Topoisomerase II inhibitors

Aamsacrine	Etoposide
Daunorubicin[a]	Idarubicin[a]
Doxorubicin[a]	Mitoxantrone
Epirubicin[a]	

(continued)

TABLE 1.7 (continued)

Cytotoxic antibiotics	
Bleomycin	Dactinomycin
Mitomycin	
Anti-microtubule drugs	
Cabazitaxel	Vincristine
Docetaxel	Vindesine
Paclitaxel	Vinorelbine
Vinblastine	

[a]May also be classified as cytotoxic antibiotics and anthracyclines

not one but two alkyl groups, and are termed bifunctional alkylating agents. The molecular distance between the two alkyl groups is such that they can each bind to a guanine base on the strands on the DNA chain where a turn in the helix brings them close together. In this way the alkylating agents form bridges, or cross-linkages, between the DNA strands which prevent them from separating at the time of DNA replication prior to cell division. In addition at those points in the DNA chain where separation does occur the alkylating agents will attach to any free guanine bases and prevent them from acting as templates for the formation of new DNA (this is a major mode of action for monofunctional alkylating agents, containing only one alkyl group, which are not able to form cross-linkages). In this way DNA replication, and hence subsequent cell division, are inhibited.

The alkylating agents can be grouped into a number of classes based on their chemical properties, and these are shown in Table 1.8.

Platinum Analogues

Cisplatin was developed following the observation, in 1965, that passing an electric current between platinum electrodes in nutrient broth inhibited the growth of bacteria. As a result cisplatin was developed, which is a complex of chlorine and

TABLE 1.8 Classification of commonly used cytotoxic alkylating agents

Nitrogen mustards

Bendamustine	Melphalan
Chlorambucil	Nitrogen mustard
Cyclophosphamide	
Ifosfamide	

Nitrosoureas

Carmustine	Lomustine

Alkylalkanesulfonates

Busulfan	Treosulfan

Aziridines

Mitomycin[a]	

Tetrazines

Dacarbazine[b]	Temozolomide[b]
Procarbazine[b]	

[a]Also classed as a cytotoxic antibiotic
[b]Monofunctional alkylating agents

ammonia ions with platinum. Following intracellular activation cisplatin forms cross linkages with DNA, mainly by attacking the N-7 moiety of the guanine, thus acting like a bifunctional alkylating agent. Indeed, in some classifications, the platinum compounds are classed as alkylating agents.

Following the discovery of cisplatin analogues have been produced, of which the two in common use are carboplatin and oxaliplatin, and further similar drugs are currently under development.

Antimetabolites

The antimetabolites were the second family of cytotoxics to be discovered and were first used in the Unites States in the late 1940s. They work as follows: before a cell can divide it must build up large reserves of nucleic acid and protein.

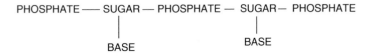

FIGURE 1.7 The structure of the DNA chain. The sugar is deoxyribose, and the bases are the pyrimidines, cytosine and thymine, and the purines, guanine and adenine

For this synthesis to take place various metabolites must be present to form the subunits from which the larger molecules will be built and enzymes must be available to achieve the synthesis. The antimetabolites may either be chemical analogues of the essential subunits, which then get incorporated into DNA in their place, making faulty DNA which prevents successful cell division, or they may be inhibitors of vital enzymes (see Figs. 1.7 and 1.8).

To understand the way the individual cytotoxic antimetabolites work it might be helpful to recap on two bits of basic cell biology: the composition of DNA and the importance of folic acid. DNA is made up of thousands of subunits called nucleotides, and each nucleotide has three components: a phosphate group; a five carbon (pentose) sugar, deoxyribose; and a nitrogen containing base. The base may be one of two purines (adenine or guanine) or pyrimidines (cytosine or thymine). Folic acid is a vitamin essential for normal cell growth. After a number of enzymatic conversions in the body it appears in its biologically active form as folinic acid. Folinic acid is an essential co-enzyme in the synthesis of purines and pyrimidines. The second stage in the conversion of folic acid to folinic acid is the transformation of dihydrofolate to tetrahydrofolate. This transformation is carried out by the enzyme dihydrofolate reductase.

The commonly used antimetabolites can be placed into three groups: those which inhibit the conversion of folic acid to folinic acid (and hence inhibit purine and pyrimidine synthesis), those which interfere with purine synthesis, and those which interfere with pyrimidine synthesis. The groups are as follows:

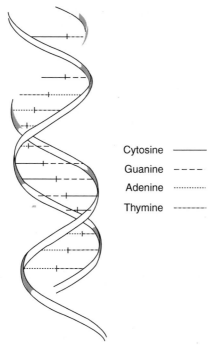

Cytosine ⎯⎯⎯

Guanine ⎯ ⎯ ⎯

Adenine ⋯⋯⋯⋯⋯

Thymine ⎯⎯⎯⎯⎯

FIGURE 1.8 The DNA complex. Two DNA chains are linked in a spiral structure by hydrogen bonds between base pairs. These bonds are highly specific: adenine can only unite with thymine and guanine can only unite with cytosine

Drugs inhibiting folinic acid production: methotrexate, pemetrexed, and raltitrexed.

Drugs interfering with purine synthesis: mercaptopurine, thioguanine, fludarabine, cladribine, hydroxyurea and pentostatin.

Drugs interfering with pyrimidine synthesis: fluorouracil, capecitabine, gemcitabine, cytaribine, and tegafur with uracil.

Leucovorin (calcium folinate, folinic acid) is an interesting compound in relation to the antimetabolites, in that it acts to both increase the efficacy of fluorouracil and reduce the toxicity of methotrexate. The active metabolites of fluorouracil work by inhibiting the enzyme thymidylate synthase, but bind only relatively weakly with this enzyme. Leucovorin strengthens this binding, and so prolongs the duration of fluorouracil's anticancer activity. The combination of fluorouracil and leucovorin has been used mainly in colorectal cancer where it has result in a virtual doubling of response rates compared to fluorouracil alone. By contrast methotrexate acts by inhibiting folinic acid synthesis, and so, following administration of high doses of the drug, any unacceptable toxicity can be arrested by giving intravenous or oral supplements of leucovorin.

Topoisomerase Inhibitors

Topoisomerase I and II are enzymes which help regulate DNA structure. Inhibition of these enzymes leads to single, or double, strand breakages in the DNA chain.

The topoisomerase I inhibitors in general use are irinotecan and topotecan. The topoisomerase II inhibitors include etoposide, doxorubicin, epirubicin, idarubicin, daunorubicin, mitoxantrone and amsacrine. Daunorubicin, doxorubicin, epirubicin and idarubicin are anthracyclines and they also act by intercalating with the DNA. This means that they sit within various parts of the DNA double helix, rather like a key in a lock, where their presence distorts the DNA template preventing the synthesis of nucleic acid.

Cytotoxic Antibiotics

In 1940 the actinomycin antibiotics were first produced from cultures of the soil bacteria actinomycetes. Although actinomycins did have antibacterial activity they were considered too toxic for human use. Subsequent research produced Dactinomycin which proved to be an effective cytotoxic. Over the following decades a number of other cytotoxics were produced from bacterial cultures and became known collectively as cytotoxic antibiotics. As more became known about their precise modes of action it became clear that some agents overlapped with other groups of cytotoxics, for example the anthracyclines were also topoisomerase II inhibitors, pentostatin was an antimetabolite, and mitomycin had alkylating activity. Other cytotoxic antibiotics have different modes of action: dactinomycin binds to DNA and prevents DNA transcription, it also causes DNA damage by free radical formation. Bleomycin also causes DNA fragmentation by free radical formation (free radicals are highly reactive molecules with unpaired electrons).

Anti-microtubule Drugs

In the past, infusions of the leaves of the garden periwinkle plant, vinca rosea, were used in folk medicine as a treatment for diabetes. In the 1950s researchers in North America tested these infusions looking, looking for a hypoglycaemic action. Instead they discovered that the plant extracts caused leucopenia. Following these observations two alkaloids were extracted from the periwinkle plant: vincristine, and vinblastine, which have subsequently proved to be valuable cytotoxic agents. Latterly vindesine and vinorelbine have been added to the family of vinca alkaloids.

In 1967 researchers in the United States, working on extracts of the bark of the Pacific yew tree, discovered the taxane cytotoxic, paclitaxel. Subsequently a second, semi-synthetic, taxane docetaxel was produced, based on an extract the needles of the European yew tree. They have now been joined by another semi-synthetic agent: cabazitaxel.

These drugs are all anti-microtubule cytotoxics. During the metaphase of mitosis, the daughter chromosomes are arranged on the cell spindle, before separating to form the two new cells. The cell spindle is formed by the protein tubulin. The antimicrotubule cytotoxics react with tubulin in one of two ways: the vinca alkaloids prevent the formation of the spindle, and the taxanes stabilise, or freeze, the spindle so that the process of mitosis cannot proceed further. In both cases, cell death results. Because of their action on the spindle these drugs are also often called cell spindle poisons.

A Note on Liposomal Formulations of Cytotoxic Drugs

Liposomes are spherical vesicles formed by a membrane made up of phospholipids and cholesterol. It is possible to encapsulate drugs within liposomes. In some instances the liposomes may also be coated by polyethylene glycol (PEG), and this is known as a pegylated liposomal formulation. In the body the liposomal coating is broken down by enzymatic degradation, or attack by macrophages, to release the drug.

The possible advantages of this liposomal formulation for cytotoxic agents are that it might prolong their circulation time before they are metabolised or excreted, it might increase their entrapment in cancers, and may reduce their access to normal cells. These effects have the potential to increase the efficacy and reduce the toxicity of the drugs.

At present in the UK doxorubicin is the only liposomally formulated cytotoxic to have been licensed, and is available in a liposomal and pegylated liposomal version. Both these formulations appear to offer a reduced risk of cardiotoxicity and cause less soft-tissue damage if the drug is extravasated, however hypersensitivity reactions and hand-foot syndrome (painful skin eruptions) are more common.

Liposomal formulations of the taxanes are also under evaluation. Docetaxel and taxotere are both difficult to get into solution and the additives necessary to do this are the agents responsible for the allergic reactions commonly seen with these agents. The liposomal formulation offers an alternative way of delivering these agents which may overcome the problem of hypersensitivity reactions for these drugs.

Suggestion for Further Reading

Park JW. Liposome-based drug delivery in breast cancer treatment. Breast Cancer Res. 2002;4:95–9.

The Development of Cytotoxic Therapy

Unlike many of the drugs we have mentioned earlier in this chapter cytotoxics have no ability to distinguish between cancer cells and normal cells. They will attack the process of cell division indiscriminately, and this causes many of their side effects, which are due to the direct damage of normal cells.

During the 1950s, more cytotoxics became available, and it was realized that different drugs interfered with the process of cell division in different ways. The logical way forward was to combine drugs with different modes of action in order to maximize cell kill, by hitting the mitotic process from a number of different directions. The only problem was that this dramatically increased toxicity, because of the corresponding increase in damage to normal cells.

The solution came with a rescheduling of the way treatment was delivered. This took advantage of the fact that cancer cells, being biologically abnormal, are much slower than normal cells in repairing injury. Normal cells could make good the damage done by cytotoxics far more rapidly than cancer cells. Previously, most cytotoxic treatments had been given continuously, and toxicity was dose-limiting. The breakthrough concept of the mid-1960s was to give the treatment intermittently. So, if a high dose of a number of cytotoxics was given on a particular day (Day 1) then within 2–3 weeks the normal cells would have recovered but the cancer cells would still be struggling to repair the damage done. So if a second dose was given on, say, Day 21 or Day 28, normal cell recovery would be complete, but the cancer cells would be hit again before they had recovered, and so would be further damaged. By giving more courses, at the same interval, normal cell integrity could be maintained, whilst the cancer cells were progressively killed off. This is the principal of intermittent combination cytotoxic chemotherapy, and it underpinned the great successes of cytotoxic therapy during the 1960s and 1970s.

Incidentally radiotherapy also works by interfering with mitosis (by forming free radicals which damage DNA in the nucleus).

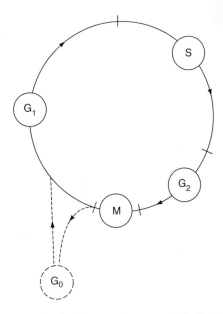

FIGURE 1.9 The cell cycle. G_0 are cells not actively dividing, G_1 is the first resting phase, S is the synthetic phase during which the cell's DNA content doubles, G_2 is the second resting, or pre-mitotic phase, and M is mitosis when the cell divides

And, like cytotoxic therapy ionising radiations also cannot distinguish between normal and cancer cells. Once again the differences in repair capacity between normal and malignant cells come into play, but in this case radiation injury can be made good by normal cells in a matter of a few hours, rather than days or weeks, and so radiotherapy doses are usually given at daily intervals, rather than with the gap of several weeks needed for normal cell recovery with cytotoxic therapy.

Cytotoxic Drugs and the Cell Cycle

In the mid-1960s it was discovered that different cytotoxic drugs affected cells in the cell cycle in different ways (see Fig. 1.9). Only one cytotoxic was found to affect cells in the resting Go stage (as well as all other phases of the cell cycle), this was

TABLE 1.9 Cell cycle phase specific drugs

G$_1$ phase-specific
Asparaginase
S phase-specific
Antimetablites
Anthracyclines
G$_2$ phase-specific
Bleomycin
Topoisomerase 1 inhibitors
M phase-specific
Vinca alkaloids
Etoposide
Taxanes

nitrogen mustard. Many drugs were shown to attack cells at all active phases of the cell cycle. Because they only attack cells which are actually in the cell cycle (as opposed to being in the resting Go stage), these are called cycle-specific drugs. They include: the alkylating agents and the platinum drugs. Some other drugs only attack cells during certain phases of the cell cycle. These are called cell cycle phase-specific, or phase-dependant drugs (see Table 1.9).

During the 1970s oncologists tried to exploit these differences by designing drug combinations and treatment schedules based on cell cycle theory. At the end of the day clinical trials showed absolutely no benefit from these complex drug regimens, and they fell out of favour. These days little or no attention is paid to cell cycle kinetics in the design of drug combinations and treatment schedules. So this whole question is really only of historic interest.

Tumour Kinetics: Adjuvant Therapy

With the start of uncontrolled mitosis the cancer has now begun to grow. In the 1960s Howard Skipper, a tumour biologist working in Birmingham, Alabama, discovered that injecting a single leukaemic cell into an immune-suppressed mouse could lead to a fatal leukaemia, showing that cancerous changes in just one cell were sufficient to be lethal. So, one cancer cell divides to become two, two divide to become four, and so on.

After some 30 cell divisions, or cell doublings, our cancer will contain about 1,000 million cells, and form a swelling approximately 1 cm in diameter (see Fig. 1.10). This is about the smallest size at which most cancers can be detected clinically, by physical examination or radiological imaging. After about another ten doublings the cancer will have achieved a lethal tumour burden and the host will die.

Although tumour growth tends to slow with time, as the intervals between doublings gradually increases, these figures still mean that for a large part of its natural history a cancer will be completely clinically undetectable: tumour masses containing tens of millions of cancer cells may be present that will not be revealed by the even the most careful examination or the most detailed CT or MRI scans.

This explains why someone can have an operation to remove a primary cancer, and appear to be free of all traces of the disease, yet still relapse with widespread secondary disease, with multiple bone, or liver, or lung metastases, a matter of months or years later. Those secondary cancers did not develop after the primary was removed, they were there at the time of the original operation, but were simply too small to be detectable.

In the 1960s this appreciation of basic tumour kinetics coincided with the major improvements in treatment of a number of advanced, metastatic, cancers as result of intermittent combination cytotoxic chemotherapy. Building on these developments a number of experts put forward a new concept: if cytotoxic chemotherapy could reduce large tumour volumes might it not be even more effective against small, microscopic foci of cancer, so that if one could identify patients who were at risk of harbouring these occult metastases after surgery for a primary cancer, and if one gave them

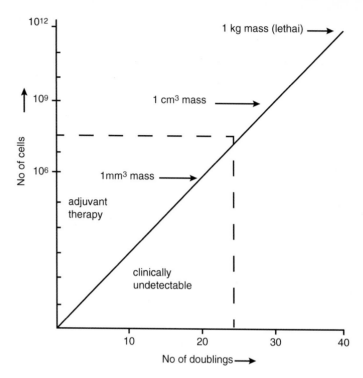

FIGURE I.IO Tumour cell population and the limit of clinical detection. As the tumour grows its growth rate slows as it begins to outgrow its blood supply and more cells move into the G_0 phase of the cell cycle

chemotherapy, could that then kill off those potentially lethal secondary cancers, and cure them?

This was put to the test in breast cancer. The presence of cancer in one or more of the axillary lymph nodes was taken as an indicator that there was a risk of spread elsewhere in the body, and clinical trials were established where women who had node-positive disease were randomized to receive either no further treatment or systemic therapy, with either cytotoxic drugs or hormonal agents. These trials rapidly showed that giving drug treatment dramatically reduced relapse rates and improved overall survival. The case for introducing systemic therapy for selected patients in the treatment of the early stages of breast cancer was proven.

This approach of giving treatment to people who are at risk of harbouring microscopic metastases after their primary treatment, even though they have no clinical evidence of disease, is called adjuvant therapy. Over the last 30 years, following the pioneering work in breast cancer, adjuvant therapy now forms a routine part of the management of a number of major cancers.

Although the introduction of adjuvant therapy has improved the outcomes in a number of cancers it is important to remember that this is a treatment of a risk, not a certainty. As the residual cancer that is being treated is, by definition, undetectable, it is impossible to know whether it is there or not, all one can say is that because of the features of their primary cancer that particular individual has a *probability* of still harbouring occult metastases. This means that in any group of individuals given adjuvant treatment a number will already have been cured by their initial surgery, or radiotherapy, and will be receiving their systemic therapy completely unnecessarily.

A further point about adjuvant therapy, which many patients find hard to understand, is that because there is no detectable or measurable disease at the outset, then there is no short-term way of knowing whether or not the treatment has worked. Doing scans, x-rays or blood tests at the end of systemic adjuvant therapy won't give the answer, and the only way of knowing if treatment has been successful is if the patient is alive and disease-free some 5–10 years later.

Gene Analysis and Treatment Selection

Historically progress in systemic cancer therapy has come from the discovery of new drugs, or developing new ways of exploiting existing therapies. The problems of patient selection, touched on in the previous section on adjuvant therapy, have been largely overlooked but are now coming into sharper focus. Unlike antibiotic therapy, where laboratory testing can be done to identify the appropriate drug treatment no 'culture and sensitivity' test has ever been successfully developed for cancers (despite countless attempts to do so). However, progress in technology based around gene analysis are offering the possibility that this may soon change.

In recent years laboratory methods have been developed that allow tissue samples to be rapidly analysed for the presence of thousands of different genes. The two techniques used to do this are called DNA microassay (or gene array assay) and real time reverse transcriptase polymerase chain reaction (RT-RTPCR) analysis.

Cancers are made up of abnormal cells and these cells contain abnormal patterns of genes. Even with the same type of cancer different patients will have different patterns of abnormal genes in their cancer cells.

It has always been recognised that individual cancers can behave quite differently. For example, two women may both have early breast cancer, and their tumours may look very similar under the microscope, but one might have very aggressively, growing and spreading rapidly, whilst the other might grow much more slowly.

The way these different cancers behave is controlled by their genes. Research using gene expression profiling is currently being used to study cancers to see if a high risk gene signature can be identified. This is a particular pattern of abnormal genes which means that the particular cancer is likely to behave more aggressively.

Some progress has been made in breast cancer and lung cancer in discovering high risk gene signatures. But this process is still at an early stage of development and gene expression profiling is still very much at the research stage.

The hope is that in years to come it may be a more routine process and may not only help in deciding whether a cancer is more or less aggressive, but might actually help in deciding what the best treatment for that cancer might be.

Suggestions for Further Reading

Espinosa E, Vara JAF, Navarro IS, et al. Gene profiling in breast cancer: time to move forward. Cancer Treat Rev. 2011;37:416–21.
Nannini M, Pantaleo MA, Astolfi A, et al. Gene expression profiling in colorectal cancer using microarray technologies: results and perspectives. Cancer Treat Rev. 2009;35:201–9.
Reis-Filho JS, Puztai L. Gene expression profiling in breast cancer: classification, prognostication and prediction. Lancet. 2011;378: 1812–23.

Bone Modifying Agents: Bisphosphonates and Denosumab

Although there is some laboratory evidence that the bisphosphonates may have a direct effect on cancer cells their main role in oncology is as a supportive therapy. They alter bone metabolism, their net effect being inhibition of osteoclast activity, leading to a reduction in bone resorption, and hence bone strengthening. This has led to their evaluation in people who have, or are at risk of developing, skeletal involvement from their cancer. In the last few years the bisphosphonates have been joined by the monoclonal antibody denosumab (Prolia) which acts in a different way to inhibit osteoclast activity.

Bone modifying agents have been most extensively studied in multiple myeloma, breast and prostate cancer. In people with multiple myeloma, and those with bone secondaries from breast or prostate cancer clinical trials show that they reduce the risk of pathological fractures and malignant hypercalcaemia and delay the onset of skeletal complications. The need for palliative radiotherapy and orthopaedic surgery is also reduced, but the risk of spinal cord compression is not affected. In multiple myeloma there is clear evidence that bisphosphonates also help with pain control, but this is less certain in breast and prostate cancer. Despite these various benefits the use of bone modifying agents does not improve overall survival in any of these patient groups.

TABLE 1.10 Bisphosphonates used in cancer care

Drug	Formulation
Disodium pamidronate	Intravenous
Ibandronic acid	Oral
Sodium clodronate	Oral
Zoledronic acid	Intravenous

At the present time bone modifying agents form part of the routine management of patients with multiple myeloma (except for those with the indolent, or smouldering, form of the disease). The extent to which they are used in people who have bone secondaries from breast or prostate cancer is variable, but they are increasingly being recommended in guidelines. It has also been suggested that bisphosphonates may have a role in adjuvant therapy for early breast cancer, reducing the risk of bone involvement and increasing survival, but recent clinical trial results have failed to confirm this. However a study looking at denosumab in men with prostate cancer has suggested it may delay the onset of bone metastases by 4 months or more, although overall survival was not affected.

Bisphosphonates are available in oral and intravenous formulations (see Table 1.10) and denosumab is administered subcutaneously. The optimum duration of therapy has still to be defined, but the usual practice is for the drugs to be given until there is clear evidence that they are no longer effective. Side effects include gastrointestinal disturbance (nausea, diarrhoea or constipation) which is more likely with oral dosing, fevers, and hypocalcaemia, which are more likely with intravenous therapy. An uncommon, but severe, complication is osteonecrosis of the jaw. This affects between 1% and 2% of patients receiving intravenous zoledronic acid or pamidronate for more than 18 months and up to 5% of those receiving denosumab; it is more likely in people with pre-existing dental problems or those requiring major dental work during treatment, and it is recommended that anyone undergoing bisphosphonate therapy should have a careful dental examination prior to treatment so that any dental problems can be corrected before starting the drugs. There has also been conflicting evidence about the risk of oesophageal cancer. If this does occur it only affects fewer than 1 in 1,000 patients and is associated with prolonged use of the drugs (for more than 5 years) and so is of little relevance in the context of oncological treatment. Atrial fibrillation and flutter may also occur in about 4% of patients with bisphosphonates but seldom cause clinical problems.

Suggestions for Further Reading

Bilezikian JP. Osteonecrosis of the jaw – do bisphosphonates pose a risk? N Engl J Med. 2006;355:2278–81.

Body J-J. Bisphosphonates for malignancy-related bone disease: current status, future developments. Support Care Cancer. 2006; 14:408–18.

Cardwell CR, Abnet CC, Cantwell MM, et al. Exposure to oral bisphosphonates and risk of esophageal cancer. JAMA. 2010;304:657–63.

Coleman RE, Marshall H, Cameron D, et al. Breast-cancer adjuvant therapy with zoledronic acid. N Engl J Med. 2011;365:1396–1405.

Erichsen R, Christiansen CF, Frøslev T, et al. Intravenous bisphosphonate therapy and atrial fibrillation/flutter risk in cancer patients: a nationwide cohort study. Br J Cancer. 2011;105:881–3.

Smith MR, Saad F, Coleman R, et al. Denosumab and bone-metastasis-free survival in men with castration-resistant prostate cancer: results of a phase 3, randomised, placebo-controlled trial. Lancet. 2012;379:39–46.

Van Poznak C, Temin S, Yee GC, et al. American Society of Clinical Oncology Executive Summary of the Clinical Practice Guideline Update on the role of bone-modifying agents in metastatic breast cancer. J Clin Oncol. 2011;29:1221–7.

Chemoprevention

To bring this chapter full circle it is reasonable to pose the question: if drugs can be used to treat cancer can they also be used to prevent it? As far as the cytotoxics are concerned, side effects preclude their use in this situation but hormonal approaches have been explored in breast cancer and other drugs have been evaluated in prostate and bowel cancer.

A number of clinical trials have been carried out randomising women who have been assessed on the basis of their family history as being at risk of developing breast cancer to receive either tamoxifen or a placebo. The results of individual trials differ but a meta-analysis has revealed that overall giving tamoxifen reduces the risk of breast cancer development by up to 40%. Despite this apparent good news there are some uncertainties about these results: the risk reduction only applies to ER+ cancers, and the women are exposed to the side effects of tamoxifen, including an increased risk of thromboembolic phenomena and endometrial cancer, furthermore no study has yet shown an overall increase in survival as a result of giving tamoxifen. Other studies have explored the use of raloxifene – a selective oestrogen receptor modifier used to treat osteoporosis, but not breast cancer, which may be as effective as tamoxifen but without some of its side effects, including the risk of endometrial cancer and a lower risk of thromboembolic complications. These have shown similar results to tamoxifen but only in postmenopausal women. Different parts of the world have reached different conclusions about these results: in the United States guidelines have been formulated for the use of tamoxifen and raloxifene in breast cancer prevention whereas in Britain no such recommendations have been made.

The US guidelines note that trials of aromatase inhibitors for breast cancer prevention in postmenopausal women are underway and at least one of these has recently reported a 65% reduction in breast cancer risk so these agents may become increasingly important in breast cancer prevention in the future.

Another condition where there has been considerable interest in chemoprevention is prostate cancer. Clinical trials have looked at the use of two drugs: finasteride and dutasteride. These both inhibit the enzyme 5α-reductase which is involved in testosterone metabolism and hence reduce circulating androgen levels. They are usually used in benign prostatic hypertrophy where they lead to shrinkage of the gland and relief of obstructive symptoms. The results showed that giving these agents for 4–7 years to men over 50 reduced the incidence of prostate cancer by 22–25%. In 2009 guidelines were actually issued in the USA suggesting that 5α-reductase inhibitors could be considered for prostate cancer prevention in men over 50. However there appeared to relatively little interest in their use and at the end of 2010 the US Food and Drugs Administration refused both drugs a licence for use in this indication. The main reasons for this refusal were a concern that in the finasteride study although overall numbers of prostate cancer had been reduced men taking the drug had seen an increased frequency of more aggressive forms of the disease, and in the dutasteride trial the reduction in numbers had been seen only in more indolent cancers which might well not have needed treatment anyway.

A different approach to chemoprevention that is generating interest is the use of aspirin. Aspirin inhibits the enzyme cyclooxygenase (COX) which leads to a reduction in prostaglandin levels, it also promotes apoptosis and inhibits angiogenesis, all these actions have an anticancer potential. There is growing evidence from epidemiological studies that taking aspirin for a number of years can reduce the risk of cancer developing, particularly colorectal cancer. However, there are uncertainties about the dose of the drug and duration of it needs to be taken in order to have an effect. Also there are concerns about potential side effects from long-term aspirin administration, such as gastrointestinal bleeding and perforation. For these reasons there are currently no moves to promote aspirin use as a form of chemoprevention in the general population but there is growing evidence that it should be used as a prophylactic measure in people who are known to carry genetic mutations which predispose to the development of bowel cancer.

Suggestions for Further Reading

Andriole GL, Bostwick DG, Brawley OW, et al. Effect of dutasteride on the risk of prostate cancer. N Engl J Med. 2010;362:1192–202.

Chan T, Lippman SM. Aspirin and colorectal cancer prevention in Lynch syndrome. Lancet. 2011;378:2051–2.

Cuzick J, DeCensi A, Arun B, et al. Preventive therapy for breast cancer: a consensus statement. Lancet Oncol. 2011;12:496–503.

Goss PE, Ingle JN, Ales-Martinez JE, et al. Exemestane for breast cancer prevention in postmenopausal women. N Engl J Med. 2011;364:2381–91.

Langley RE, Burdett S, Tierney JF, et al. Aspirin and cancer: has aspirin been overlooked as an adjuvant therapy. Br J Cancer. 2011;105:1107–113.

Mellon JK. The finasteride prostate cancer prevention trial (PCPT) – what have we learned? Eur J Cancer. 2005;41:2016–22.

Visvanathan K, Chlebowski RT, Hurley P, et al. American Society of Clinical Oncology clinical practice guideline update on the use of pharmacologic interventions including tamoxifen, raloxifene, and aromatase inhibition for breast cancer risk reduction. J Clin Oncol. 2009;27:3235–58.

Chapter 2
Practical Aspects of Cancer Chemotherapy

Drug Dosing

For the last 50 years most cytotoxics have been prescribed in relation to the patient's body surface area. The surface area is calculated from their height and weight, either by the use of nomograms or pre-programmed calculators or computers. The same principle is used for some, but not all, of the newer targeted therapies but, by contrast, hormonal treatments are almost always prescribed in standard doses that are the same for everybody.

The original rationale for prescribing cytotoxics on the basis of body surface area came from the realisation that there was only a narrow therapeutic window between unacceptable toxicity and efficacy for many of these agents: give too large a dose and the patient could well die from side-effects, give too small a dose and the drug would be ineffective against the cancer, and often the margin for error was small. So there was a need to individualise cytotoxic dosing. Many different factors may influence someone's response to a given dose of a drug, including their age, sex, their body size, any co-morbidities, liver and kidney function which might affect drug metabolism and excretion, and other drugs they are receiving. Measuring and assessing all these parameters for every patient is not generally practical and research in the late 1950s indicated that, for cytotoxics, adjusting the dose of drug according to the patient's surface area, was an

T. Priestman, *Cancer Chemotherapy in Clinical Practice*,
DOI 10.1007/978-0-85729-727-3_2,
© Springer-Verlag London 2012

acceptable surrogate in most instances. So the convention was established of prescribing cytotoxics on the basis of mg/m^2 surface area.

One cytotoxic that is the exception to this rule is carboplatin. The toxicity of carboplatin is closely related to its concentration in the blood over time, which in turn relates to its clearance by the kidney. The dose of carboplatin is therefore worked out by a formula, the Calvert formula, which takes account of a target blood/time level (the area under the curve, or AUC) and renal function (in terms of the glomerular filtration rate, GFR). The target AUC is usually either 5 or 7 mg/ml/min (depending on whether the patient has had previous treatment or not). The GFR may either be measured directly by the 51Cr-EDTA method or calculated by formulae such as those of Cockroft-Gault, Jellieff or Chatelet, based on measurements of serum creatinine. The Calvert formula is: $\text{dose} = \text{AUC} \times (\text{GFR} + 25)$.

Suggestions for Further Reading

Gurney H. Developing a new framework for dose calculation. J Clin Oncol. 2006;24:1489–90.

Kaestner SA, Sewell GJ. Chemotherapy dosing part I: scientific basis for current practice and use of body surface area. Clin Oncol. 2007;19:23–37.

Kaestner SA, Sewell GJ. Chemotherapy dosing part II: alternative approaches and future prospects. Clin Oncol. 2007;19:99–107.

Drug Delivery

Venous Lines

Historically, having a course of chemotherapy involved multiple venepunctures, both for all the blood tests that needed to be done and for giving the drugs themselves. This had disadvantages from a patient point of view – repeated discomfort, needle phobia – and practically – the difficulty of finding 'a good vein'. Increasingly nowadays using a venous line offers an alternative. The line is a fine hollow silicone rubber catheter, which is inserted into a vein, and stays in place throughout the time of the chemotherapy. Two types of line are used: a central line, or a PICC (peripherally inserted central catheter) line. Central lines are also sometimes known by the names of the manufacturers of the lines, the two main ones being Hickman and Groshong.

The central line is inserted through the skin just below the collar bone. It is then tunneled for a distance subcutaneously before entering into the subclavian vein, and then threaded through this until its tip lies in the superior vena cava, just above the heart. The subcutaneous tunneling of the line helps reduce the risk of infection in the line. A PICC line is inserted through one of the large veins near the bend of the elbow, and threaded along this, through the subclavian vein and into the superior vena cava.

PICC lines are cheaper and simpler to insert than central lines but are usually only suitable for short term therapies over a maximum of 6–8 weeks, whereas central lines can stay in place for a year or more. Also many oncologists feel that drugs which are likely to cause irritation to the veins, such as anthracycline cytotoxics (doxorubicin and epidubicin), and fluorouracil, are not suitable for use with PICC lines.

Once in place, the line can be used for taking blood tests, and for giving all the drugs that would normally have to be injected into a vein, or given through a drip. Putting in the line is a simple procedure. Placing a PICC line can be done as an out-patient and does not need a general anaesthetic. The skin where the line is to be inserted is numbed with local anaesthetic, and threading the line through the veins is usually quite painless, so there shouldn't be much discomfort while this is being done. The insertion only takes a few minutes and is followed immediately by a chest x-ray immediately to check that the tip of the line is in the correct position. Putting in a central line is very similar, but sometimes this may be done with a short general anaesthetic rather than a local anaesthetic.

TABLE 2.1 Complications of central venous line insertion

Immediate – at the time of insertion	
Cardiac arrhythmia	13%[a]
Arterial puncture	2%
Tip in wrong position	2%
Pneumothorax	1%
Haemorrhage	1%
Late – following insertion	
Infection	4–40%
Thrombosis	
Symptomatic	5–40%
Asymptomatic	5–60%
Migration of catheter tip	5%
Fracture of catheter	3%

[a]%ages indicate the frequency of these complications, but their incidence varies widely in different series

Once the line is in place it is important that it doesn't get blocked. To prevent this it will have to be flushed through on a regular basis. Typical schedules for this are a weekly flush with 50 iu of heparin in 5 ml of 0.9% saline once weekly, or 500 iu heparin in 5 ml saline once monthly, or simply regular flushes with saline. This may be done by chemotherapy nurses or by the patients themselves.

Normally lines are relatively trouble-free. The most common problems that do occur are shown in Table 2.1. Of the immediate problems, which occur at the time of line insertion, the arrhythmias although the commonest are not usually clinically significant. The reported incidence of late complications varies enormously in different series. When thrombosis occurs it may be of one of three types:

• fibrin sheath formation around the catheter: this is only troublesome if it affects the tip of the catheter, leading to complete or partial obstruction

- intraluminal thrombosis which may either go undetected or may lead to blockage of the catheter
- blood vessel thrombosis: effectively a deep vein thrombosis in the vessel around the catheter.

Apart from possible catheter obstruction thrombosis may lead to pulmonary embolism which possibly complicates 5% of thrombotic episodes, or the phlebitis may result in venous distension and swelling of the ipsilateral arm, which may complicate up to 10% of thromboses.

Over the years improvements in catheter design and the use of low thrombotic materials in their manufacture have reduced the risk of thrombosis but it does remain a common problem and this has led to the suggestion that giving people with central venous lines prophylactic anticoagulant therapy may be beneficial. However, the evidence from clinical trials does not really support this and it is not usually recommended.

Removing lines is normally very simple. It is done in the out-patient clinic, with just a local anaesthetic to avoid any discomfort, and only takes a few minutes.

Suggestions for Further Reading

British Committee for Standards in Haematology. BCSH guidelines on the insertion and management of central venous access devices in adults. 2006. www.bcshguidelines.com.

Rosovsky RP, Kuter DJ. Intravenous access and catheter management. In: Chabner BA, Longo DL, editors. Cancer chemotherapy and biotherapy. 5th ed. Philadelphia: Lippincott, Williams and Wilkins; 2011. p. 746–58.

Young AM, Billingham LJ, Begum G, et al. Warfarin prophylaxis in cancer patients with central venous catheters (WARP): an open-label randomised trial. Lancet. 2009;373:567–74.

Implantable Ports

Implantable ports (which are also known as portocaths) are a variation on venous lines. The line is placed in a similar way, but instead of the end of it coming out on the skin, it ends in a subcutaneous port. This is a small soft plastic bubble, between about 2.5 and 4 cm across, which lies just under the surface of the skin. This means it is less obvious than a central or PICC line, and appears as just a small bump under the skin. It is usually placed near the top of the front of the chest.

Like central lines, implantable ports may be inserted either as an out-patient, using a local anaesthetic, or occasionally as a day-patient, if a general anaesthetic is used. They also need regular flushing to stop them becoming blocked.

Once in place implantable ports can be used just like the venous lines: for taking blood tests, or giving chemotherapy or blood transfusions or other intravenous fluids.

Infusion Pumps

When a chemotherapy drug is given into a vein it is usual to set up an intravenous infusion, with a bag of fluid, on a drip stand, which trickles through a tube into the vein. The drug may either be given as an injection into the tubing of the drip, or it may be mixed with the fluid in the bag and run in as an infusion.

Depending on the treatment that is being given, the infusion may last for anywhere from a few minutes to a few hours. But some chemotherapy treatments require the drugs to be given into a vein over a matter of days or even weeks. For these long infusions, a portable pump can be used, along with a venous line. The pump is a battery-driven device that holds a syringe, containing the chemotherapy drug. This is attached to the end of the venous line, and very slowly the pump squeezes a trickle of the drug into the vein. Once the infusion is complete, then the pump is easily disconnected.

Pumps vary in size, but are usually little bigger than a mobile phone. They can be worn in a special 'holster', meaning that they are easy to carry around, and not very obvious. This means that treatment can continue when the patient is at home, and there should be very little effect on there normal day-to-day activities while the infusion is in progress (Figs. 2.1 and 2.2).

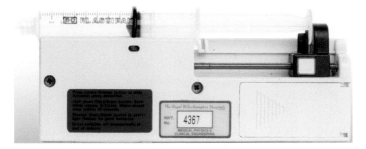

FIGURE 2.1 A battery-driven chemotherapy pump (Courtesy of Mr Simon Glazebrook, New Cross Hospital, Wolverhampton)

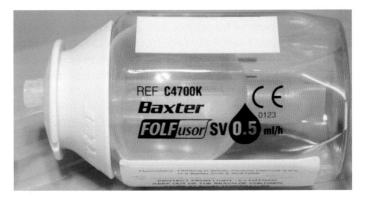

FIGURE 2.2 A disposable elastomeric infusion pump (Courtesy of Mr Simon Glazebrook, New Cross Hospital, Wolverhampton)

Epidural Chemotherapy

Very occasionally, most often with certain types of leukaemia, it may be necessary to give chemotherapy drugs via a lumbar puncture, into the space around the spinal cord, so that the drug can reach parts of the nervous system that it might not get to if it was given by an ordinary infusion into a vein. This type of treatment is called epidural chemotherapy. Unfortunately in the UK there have been a number of fatal accidents in the past as a result of this technique, when either the wrong drug, or wrong doses of a cytotoxic, were given. Because of this there are now very strict regulations and protocols governing this particular type of treatment.

Side Effects of Cancer Chemotherapy

Most chemotherapy today is still based on the use of cytotoxic drugs; hormonal treatment is important in breast and prostate cancer, and the newer targeted therapies are gaining an increasing role in cancer treatment. These different groups of drugs have very different patterns of toxicity. Because of the frequency and potential severity of their side effects the potential adverse reactions to cytotoxics will be considered in some detail in this section. In discussing these it is important to remember that patients often react differently to the same treatment. Two people can have identical chemotherapy, for the same type of cancer, and be of similar age, with a similar level of fitness, one may experience virtually no problems, whilst the other might suffer considerable side effects, and their treatment may be quite challenging.

Common Side Effects of Cytotoxic Treatment

Cytotoxic drugs interfere directly with the process of mitosis. They have no ability to distinguish between cancer cells and normal cells, and so inhibit cell division in both populations. This accounts for many of their side effects. This means that the use of cytotoxic treatment is the art of differential poisoning: killing the cancer without killing the patient. Unfortunately it is easy to get this balance wrong and people still regularly die from the side effects of cytotoxic chemotherapy. Being aware of what those side effects are, and being vigilant to detect their development as early as possible, is therefore a priority for all clinicians involved with this form of treatment.

There are many different cytotoxic drugs, and many different combinations of these drugs are used in cancer treatment. This means that the potential side effects vary considerably depending on the drugs, and the doses that are used. Having said this, there are some side effects that occur much more often than others. These include bone marrow suppression, nausea and vomiting, tiredness, alopecia, oral mucositis, and reduced fertility. A much less common but very important problem is the risk of second cancers.

Marrow Suppression

Normally the effect of a dose of chemotherapy on the bone marrow cells is temporary. The changes come on a few days after treatment, reaching a peak at about 10–14 days, and then recovering over the next week or so.

The production of white blood cells is the process most sensitive to cytotoxic inhibition; changes to the red cells and platelets generally occur more slowly, and are only likely to show up after several courses of chemotherapy (and very often are not affected at all, throughout the entire treatment). Typically, the white cell count begins to fall about 5–7 days after a dose of cytotoxics, and will reach its lowest level about 2 weeks after the treatment. The count then recovers, and will be more or less back to normal by the end of the third week. This means that there is an increased risk of infection while having chemotherapy. The combination of an infection with neutropenia is termed febrile neutropenia (in more severe cases the term neutropenic sepsis is used).

Febrile neutropenia is defined as an oral temperature >38.5°C, or two consecutive readings of >38.0°C 2 h apart and an absolute neutrophil count <0.5 × 10^9/l, or expected to fall below <0.5 × 10^9/l.

This is a common and potentially serious complication and carries an overall mortality of about 5% although in some haematological cancers this figure can rise to about 10%.

Some chemotherapy regimens are more likely than others to cause profound neutropenia (see Table 2.2). A number of

TABLE 2.2 Chemotherapy regimens associated with a greater than 20% risk of febrile neutropenia

Acronym	Drugs	Indication
AT	Doxorubicin, docetaxel	Breast cancer
CAV	Cyclophosphamide, doxorubicin, vincristine	Lung cancer
DHAP	Dexamethasone, cisplatin, cytarabine	Non-Hodgkin lymphoma
Doc	Docetaxel	Breast cancer
ESHAP	Etoposide, methylprednisolone, cisplatin, cytarabine	Non-Hodgkin lymphoma
TAC	Docetaxel, doxorubicin, cyclophosphamide	Breast cancer
Topo	Topotecan	Lung cancer
VAPEC-B	Vincristine, doxorubicin, prednisolone, etoposide, cyclophosphamide, bleomycin	Non-Hodgkin lymphoma
VelP	Vinblastine, ifosfamide, cisplatin	Germ cell (testicular cancer)

other factors have been identified which increase the risk of febrile neutropenia and these are listed in Table 2.3.

Everyone undergoing cytotoxic chemotherapy should be alerted to the risk of febrile neutropenia. They should be warned that if, at any time during treatment, they get a temperature of more than 38°C, or if they develop symptoms suggesting an infection – like shivering, a sore throat, or a cough and shortness of breath, or cystitis, or if they simply suddenly feel unwell – then they should let the hospital know immediately, so that they can attend for assessment.

Neutropenic sepsis is considered a medical emergency requiring admission to hospital. Subsequent management depends on whether the individual is thought to be at low risk or high risk of developing further complications. The Multinational Association

TABLE 2.3 Patient-related factors increasing the risk of febrile neutropenia

Pre-existing neutropenia due to disease infiltration of bone marrow or other aetiology

Age >65 years

Advanced disease stage

Presence of a central venous line

Poor performance status

Previous episodes of febrile neutropenia whilst receiving earlier chemotherapy of a similar or less dose intensity

Extensive prior chemotherapy

Previous irradiation to large volume of bone marrow

Poor nutritional status

Active infections

Increased risk of infections due to skin or gut damage

Serious co-morbidities

for Supportive Care (MASCC) index is a widely used scoring system for classifying patients as high or low risk (Table 2.4). In both instances initial management will involve antibiotic therapy which will usually be given intravenously although for some people in the low risk category oral therapy may well be possible. Each department will have its own protocol specifying which antibiotics should be used. For people in the high risk category additional measures may be needed depending on the apparent site of infection and whether or not there are complications such as dehydration, hypotension and renal failure.

For those in the low risk group the mortality is about 1% and this has led to the suggestion that selected patients might be managed on an out-patient basis but this approach remains the exception and hospital admission is the norm, although an early discharge following resolution of fever and symptomatic stabilization is often possible.

Wherever possible once someone has recovered from an episode of neutropenic sepsis the aim will be for them to

TABLE 2.4 The MASCC scoring system

Characteristic	Score
No or mild symptoms	5
Moderate symptoms	3
Severe symptoms	0
No hypotension (systolic BP >90 mmHg)	5
No chronic obstructive pulmonary disease	4
Solid tumour or lymphoma with no previous fungal infection	4
No dehydration	3
Out-patient at onset of fever	3
Age <60 years	2

Scores equal to or greater than 21 are at low risk of complications

continue their planned chemotherapy with no dose reduction. For some people this may involve the use of prophylactic antibiotics prior to and during subsequent cycles of treatment, for others the use of granulocyte colony stimulating factors (GCSF) may be considered. Once again the guidelines for using GCSF vary from country to country (in part influenced by cost considerations), and from department to department, but Table 2.5 gives a typical set of criteria in the UK.

The incidence of anaemia during chemotherapy, defined by a haemoglobin (Hb) level of <10 g/dl, is difficult to quantify, with estimates ranging from 20% to 60% of patients being affected. Clearly when the Hb level does fall below 10 g/dl symptoms will usually be fairly obvious, and treatment can be given. In the last few years, however, a number of studies have shown that patients can experience fatigue and other symptoms, when their Hb level falls to between 10 and 12 g/dl during their treatment. This a level that many clinicians would not usually consider as significantly anaemic but treatment to bring their Hb to above the 12 g/dl level has been shown to greatly improve their quality of life.

TABLE 2.5 Typical UK indications for the use of GCSF in patients receiving cytotoxic chemotherapy

GCSF may be used as either primary prophylaxis, to prevent the development of severe neutropenia, or secondary prophylaxis, to prevent recurrence of neutropenia with subsequent courses of treatment after an initial episode of neutropenic sepsis.

1. Primary Prophylaxis.

Primary prophylaxis may be considered in the following circumstances:

(i)   Patients receiving radical or adjuvant chemotherapy who are at ≥40% risk of developing neutropenic fever

(ii) Hospitalised patients receiving radical or adjuvant chemotherapy who are at ≥20% risk of developing neutropenic fever while an inpatient.

(iii) Patients aged >65 receiving radical or adjuvant chemotherapy who are at ≥20% risk of developing neutropenic fever

(iv) Patients aged >50 with significant pulmonary or cardiovascular comorbidity receiving radical or adjuvant chemotherapy who are at ≥20% risk of developing neutropenic fever

(v)   Patients aged with leukaemia or lymphoma receiving radical chemotherapy who are at ≥20% risk of developing neutropenic fever

The risk is assessed on the basis of the patient's age, tumour type, performance status, comorbidities and the likely myelotoxicity of the chosen drug regimen (see Table 2.2).

2. Secondary prophylaxis.

The use of GCSF should be considered in patients receiving curative chemotherapy for cancers where maintenance of dose intensity may improve survival. However the optimum scheduling of GCSF is not defined.

The choice of treatment for chemotherapy-induced anaemia rests between blood transfusion or the use of erythropoietic agents such as epoetin alfa (Eprex), epoetin beta (NeroRecormon) or darbepoetin alfa (Aranesp). These are all related to the hormone erythropoietin, which is produced in the kidneys and stimulates red blood cell production.

Although costly these agents were quite widely used in the past. However, more recently results from a number of studies have raised questions over the safety of these agents, suggesting they could lead to an increase in cancer growth and might cause thromboembolic complications. These concerns have led NICE in the UK to recommend that they are only used for women undergoing chemotherapy for ovarian cancer with platinum-based drugs who develop anaemia or people with severe treatment-related anaemia who are unable to have blood transfusions. The current US guidelines are slightly different, recommending that these agents should not be given to people undergoing curative chemotherapy.

Suggestions for Further Reading

De Naurois J, Novitzky-Basso I, Gill MJ, et al. Management of febrile neutropenia: ESMO clinical practice guidelines. Ann Oncol. 2010; 21 Suppl 5:v252–6.

NCCN clinical practice guidelines in oncology: cancer- and chemotherapy-induced anemia. Version 2.2012, 2011. National Comprehensive Cancer Network.

NICE technology appraisal 142. Epoetin alfa, epoetin beta and darbepoetin alfa for cancer treatment-induced anaemia. National Institute for Health and Clinical Excellence. 2008.

Smith TJ, Khatcheresian J, Lyman GH, et al. Update of recommendations for the use of white blood cell growth factors: an evidence-based clinical practice guideline. J Clin Oncol. 2006;24:3187–205.

Nausea and Vomiting

Many cytotoxic treatments result in nausea and vomiting. The nausea comes on a few hours after the drugs are given. It is usually at its worst during the first 2 days after the chemotherapy, and then settles quite quickly over another day or two. The chance of experiencing sickness, and the severity of that sickness, vary enormously with different drugs, and the commonly used agents may be classified into those at high risk of emesis (where >90% of patients are likely to be affected), moderate risk (30–90%), low risk (10–30%), and minimal risk (<10%) (see Table 2.6).

TABLE 2.6 The emetic potential of anti-cancer drugs

Minimal risk

   Bevacizumab

   Bleomycin

   Busulfan

   Cetuximab

   Chlorambucil

   Gefitinib

   Imatinib

   Fludarabine

   Rituximab

   Vinblastine

   Vincristine

   Vinorelbine

Low risk

   Bortezomib

   Cabazetaxel

   Capecitabine

   Cytarabine $<1,000$ mg/m^2

   Docetaxel

   Etoposide

   Fluorouracil

   Gemcitabine

   Methotrexate

   Mitomycin

   Mitoxantrone

   Paclitaxel

   Panitumumab

(continued)

TABLE 2.6 (continued)

Pemetrexed

Temsirolimus

Topotecan

Trastuzumab

Moderate risk

Azacitidine

Alemtuzumab

Bendamustine

Carboplatin

Clofarabine

Cyclophosphamide <1,500 mg/m^2

Cytarabine >1,000 mg/m^2

Daunorubicin[a]

Doxorubicin[a]

Epirubicin[a]

Idarubicin[a]

Ifosfamide

Irinotecan

Oxaliplatin

Procarbazine

Temozolamide

High risk

Carmustine

Cisplatin

Cyclophosphamide >1,500 mg/m^2

Dacarbazine

Dactinomycin

Nitrogen mustard

[a]These anthracyclines are high emetic risk if combined with cyclophosphamide

There is also evidence that some people are more vulnerable to chemotherapy-induced nausea and vomiting than others: women are more at risk than men, especially if they have experienced emesis during pregnancy; younger people are more at risk than older people; and a history of motion sickness means problems are more likely. A key point in managing cytotoxic emesis is to prevent it happening in the first place, so anti-emetic treatment is usually given as prophylaxis, rather than waiting for symptoms to develop. Although huge improvements have been made in the control of emesis over the last 20 years nausea can still be more difficult to prevent than vomiting.

For many years control of emesis relied on dopamine antagonists like metoclopramide (Maxolon) or domperidone (Motilium). Prevention and treatment of cytotoxic-induced emesis then improved dramatically in the 1990s with the introduction of the 5HT3 receptor antagonists, ondansetron (Zofran) and granisetron (Kytril). These were followed by the second generation drug palonosetron (Aloxi), which is the only 5HT3 receptor antagonist effective in preventing delayed emesis: sickness that comes on a day or two after chemotherapy and which is a troublesome feature of cisplatin and a number of highly emetogenic chemotherapy regimens. 5HT3 receptors, which are stimulated by serotonin (5-hydroxytryptamine) form part of both the central and peripheral pathways for the stimulation of nausea and vomiting. The effectiveness of all these drugs can be further increased by giving the steroid, dexamethasone, which is also an effective anti-emetic in its own right, at the same time.

A further development has been the introduction the neurokinin-1 (NK_1) inhibitors. These work in a different way to other anti-sickness drugs by inhibiting NK_1 receptors in the brain. These receptors are key to triggering the vomiting reflex and are stimulated by a neurotransmitter called substance P. The first NK_1 inhibitor in clinical use was aprepitant (Emend) which was followed by fosaprepitant (Emend for injection in the USA, Ivemend in Europe). The NK_1 inhibitors are especially good at preventing delayed emesis.

The protocol for anti-emetic therapy can be tailored to the risk of symptoms developing. So for minimal risk drugs treatment may not be necessary but if problems do occur then

TABLE 2.7 Advice for patients to reduce their risk of nausea

Avoid greasy, fatty or very spicy foods.

Ginger can help to ease sickness; so try nibbling a ginger biscuit or drinking ginger ale or ginger beer.

Avoid big meals, eat little and often with light bites and snacks

If you feel sick first thing in the morning, keep a couple of dry biscuits by your bed and try to eat one before you get up.

Make sure you have plenty of fresh air; keep a window open if you can, especially when cooking.

If cooking smells upset you, try to get someone else to prepare your meals, or opt for cold food, with salads and sandwiches.

Sea-bands may be helpful. These are bands that you strap on round your wrists. They are fitted with a button that gently presses on the skin over an acupressure point on the inner surface of the wrist. You can buy these sea-bands at any chemist.

metoclopramide or domperidone, starting immediately prior to chemotherapy and given tds for 4 days, should suffice. For low risk therapy a single dose of 8 mg dexamethasone 30–60 min before drug administration is recommended. For moderate risk drugs a combination of dexamethasone and a 5HT3 antagonist should be given whereas for high risk chemotherapy a three drug regimen is recommended with dexamethasone, a 5HT3 antagonist and an NK_1 inhibitor. These schedules will prevent sickness altogether, or keep it to a very low, and tolerable, level for the great majority of people.

Although 5HT3 antagonists are very effective at preventing and relieving sickness, some people do find they get side effects from them. The most common of these are constipation and headache. These can usually be relieved with a simple laxative like Senokot, or a simple painkiller like paracetemol. The NK_1 inhibitors can also cause side effects including hiccups, indigestion, diarrhea, constipation, loss of appetite and tiredness.

In addition to these pharmacological measures there are also things that patients can do themselves to help reduce the risk of nausea during chemotherapy. These are summarised in Table 2.7.

Suggestions for Further Reading

Basch E, Prestrud AA, Hesketh PJ, et al. Antiemetics: American Society of Clinical Oncology clinical practice guidelines update. J Clin Oncol. 2011;29:4189–98.
Hesketh P. Chemotherapy-induced nausea and vomiting. N Engl J Med. 2008;358:2482–94.

Tiredness or Fatigue

Profound tiredness, or fatigue, is a very common problem during chemotherapy. It is thought that four out of five people will experience fatigue on some days during their treatment, and for about one in three it will be present most of the time. Not only is there often a complete lack of energy, but the tiredness can also interfere with other things – like memory, sleeping, and sex life. It may also lead to symptoms like breathlessness and loss of appetite. The tiredness usually comes on during the first week or two of treatment, and often gets more apparent as the course of treatment continues. Once the chemotherapy is over, the sense of fatigue slowly reduces, but it can take anywhere from a month or two to more than a year before it completely disappears. Studies suggest that even a year after treatment has finished, about one in five people will still regularly have days when they feel fatigued. Generally speaking, the older the patient, the longer it takes to recover their stamina. Tiredness is also more likely if someone is having, or has recently had, other treatments, like surgery or radiotherapy.

Although it is something that affects the majority of people, doctors have been slow to realize how important this tiredness is, and have concentrated on more obvious side effects like sickness and the risk of infection. This means there has been relatively little research into the causes and treatment of chemotherapy-related fatigue. Chemotherapy itself undoubtedly does cause fatigue, but frequently there can be other factors that might make the feeling worse. These include anaemia, the presence of an infection, being clinically depressed, or being in pain. All these are things that can often readily be corrected. So if someone does complain of feeling very tired, then it is important to make sure none of these other factors are present.

Anaemia can usually be rapidly reversed by a simple blood transfusion, which can often be given as an out-patient. Even very mild levels of anaemia, with an Hb of 12 g/l or less, which would not normally be troublesome, can lead to severe tiredness in people who are having chemotherapy, and correcting this can make a big difference to how they feel. Similarly, giving antibiotics, or antifungal drugs, for an infection, or analgesics to relieve pain, or prescribing antidepressants for people who are clinically depressed, can ease their feeling of tiredness quite dramatically.

Some recent research has looked at giving the psychostimulant methylphenidate, Ritalin (used to treat attention-deficit-hyperactivity-disorder,ADHD)topeoplewithcancer-related fatigue. These were randomised controlled trials comparing Ritalin with a placebo. Although there was some improvement among the people taking Ritalin there was also an improvement for those on the placebo. Whether this was simply a 'placebo-effect' or whether it was because, since they were in a trial, people were getting more support, in the form of additional consultations, tests, and telephone interviews from specialist nurses was uncertain. At the moment these results are not strong enough to recommend Ritalin routinely but the benefit in the placebo group suggests that just identifying the problem of chemotherapy-related fatigue and taking it seriously can have a positive effect.

An important thing to remember is to reassure people that tiredness is a very common feature of chemotherapy, and it does not mean that their cancer is coming back, or getting worse, nor does it mean that things are going wrong with their treatment.

Suggestions for Further Reading

Bruera E, Yennurajalingam S. Challenge of managing cancer-related fatigue. J Clin Oncol. 2010;28:3671–2.
Hofman M, Ryan JL, Colmar D, et al. Cancer-related fatigue: the scale of the problem. Oncologist. 2007;12 Suppl 1):4–7. This supplement includes a number of interesting papers on cancer-related fatigue.

Minton O, Richardson A, Sharpe M, et al. A systematic review and meta-analysis of the pharmacological treatment of cancer-related fatigue. J Nat Cancer Inst. 2008;100:1556–66.

Mild Cognitive Impairment: Chemobrain

Whilst tiredness is a well-recognised and universally accepted side-effect of cytotoxic chemotherapy the risk of mild cognitive impairment as a result of treatment is more controversial. Although there is growing evidence for the phenomenon many oncologists remain sceptical about the existence of the problem. However, a number of studies, mostly looking at women treated for breast cancer, have reported people experiencing problems such as memory loss, difficulty in concentrating, difficulty in learning, reduced ability to multi-task and general mental 'fogginess'. These changes may appear acutely or at a later date. At the present time there are many unanswered questions about this possible toxicity: the incidence of the problem, the timing of onset, whether it is related to specific drugs and how it should be managed all remain unclear but the oncological community is increasingly accepting that the condition does exist and research is underway to try and define it more clearly.

Suggestions for Further Reading

Argyriou AA, Assimakopoulas K, Iconomou G, et al. Either called 'chemo-brain' or 'chemo-fog' the long-term chemotherapy induced cognitive decline in cancer survivors is real. J Pain Symptom Manage. 2011;41:126–39.
Wefel JC, Saleeba AK, Buzdar AV, Meyers CA. Acute and late onset cognitive dysfunction associated with chemotherapy in women with breast cancer. Cancer. 2010;116:3348–56.

Hair Loss

For many people, the idea of having chemotherapy means that you must lose your hair. Alopecia is a major problem with cytotoxic treatment but not with most other types of cancer chemotherapy. The risk of hair loss is linked directly to which cytotoxic drugs are given, with some hair loss is almost inevitable, with others it is virtually unknown (see Table 2.8). Both the incidence of hair loss and its impact on people's quality of life has frequently been underestimated by health professionals.

When hair loss occurs, it usually develops about 3–4 weeks after starting treatment. Frequently, once it starts, it can progress very rapidly, with almost complete hair loss within a day or two; with other types of treatment, it may be more a case of gradual thinning of the hair over several months. Scalp hair is the most sensitive to the effects of chemotherapy, because it grows more rapidly than hair on other parts of the body. But sometimes the drugs will cause loss of eyebrows, eyelashes, under-arm hair, and pubic hair as well. As well as warning patients about the risk of hair loss it is vital to remember to reassure them that, however much hair is lost, it will always grow back again (except occasionally in those undergoing high dose chemotherapy with a bone marrow or stem cell transplant). Normally the hair begins to reappear a month or so after the end of chemotherapy, and is back completely within 3–6 months (sometimes it even starts to grow while people are still having the drugs). Often, however, it comes back with a different colour and appearance – a grey/black, 'pepper and salt' colouring, with quite a thick texture, and a slightly curly or wavy look is very common, although these changes may be transient.

If treatment does involve drugs that carry a high risk of alopecia, the one thing that can sometimes be done to try to prevent, or reduce, this is scalp cooling. There are various types of scalp cooling, but the general principle is to chill the scalp, usually by wearing a special padded hat that contains a gel. The hat is stored in a freezer and is then strapped firmly on the patient's head about half an hour before they are due to have their drugs. It has been suggested that wetting the hair before applying the cap may increase its effectiveness but this is uncertain. They then continue to wear the hat for about half an hour after the drugs have been given. The underlying principle is that by keeping the scalp very cold the

TABLE 2.8 Cytotoxics and hair loss

Drugs which carry a high risk of total alopecia, or cosmetically significant hair loss

Cyclophosphamide	Etoposide
Dactinomycin	Ifosfamide
Daunorubicin	Irinotecan
Docetaxel	Paclitaxel
Doxorubicin	Temozolamide
Epirubicin	Vindesine

Drugs which sometimes cause noticeable hair loss, or thinning of the hair

Amsacrine	Lomustine
Bleomycin	Melphalan
Busulfan	Pemetrexed
Cytarabine	Pentostatin
Fludarabine	Topotecan
Fluorouracil	Vinblastine
Gemcitabine	Vincristine
Hydroxyurea	Vinorelbine
Idarubicin	

Drugs which rarely, or never cause hair loss

Capecitabine	Mitomycin
Carboplatin	Mitoxantrone
Carmustine	Oxaliplatin
Chlorambucil	Procarbazine
Cisplatin	Raltitrexed
Cladribine	Tegafur
Dacarbazine	Thiotepa
Mercaptopurine	Thioguanine
Methotrexate	Treosulfan

blood vessels in the scalp contract, so the blood supply to the hair follicles is reduced and they will be less affected by the circulating cytotoxics. Scalp cooling doesn't always work. For many people it will prevent or greatly reduce the amount of hair loss, but for others it has very little effect. One group of patients in whom it is often ineffective are those who have disturbed liver function, due to liver secondaries or other causes, which delays metabolism of many cytotoxic drugs, and hence maintains their concentration in the blood after the scalp cooling is complete. Some people find scalp cooling uncomfortable. The hat is very cold, and can often cause headaches and occasionally dizziness and light-headedness, so it does not suit everyone (Fig. 2.3).

There have been concerns about the use of cold caps increasing the risk of scalp metastases but there is no clear evidence for this from clinical studies. However, the use of scalp cooling is generally considered contraindicated in people with haematological cancers and malignant melanoma because of this uncertainty.

For those people who do develop alopecia the most obvious way of coping is having a wig. Most chemotherapy departments have a specially trained member of staff who can discuss the available options with and arrange a wig that meets the individual's colour and style. Alternatives to wigs include headscarves and bandanas, which allow some people to turn their hair loss into a fashion statement!

Patients often ask if there is anything that they can do to reduce the risk of hair loss, and Table 2.9 gives some useful tips.

Suggestions for Further Reading

Breed WPM, ven den Hurk CJG, Peerbooms M. Presentation, impact and prevention of chemotherapy-induced hair loss. Expert Rev Dermatol. 2011;6:109–25.

Hesketh PJ, Batchelor D, Golant M. Chemotherapy-induced alopecia: psychosocial impact and therapeutic approaches. Support Care Cancer. 2004;12:543–9.

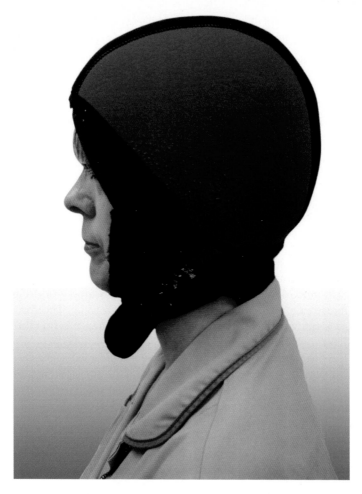

FIGURE 2.3 A typical 'cold cap' used for scalp cooling to prevent chemotherapy-induced hair loss (Courtesy of the author)

Oral Mucositis

Having a sore mouth during chemotherapy is quite common as a result of inflammation of the lining of the mouth. The chances of getting a sore mouth do vary depending on the

TABLE 2.9 Advice for patients to reduce their risk of alopecia

Avoid using heated products like curling tongs or heated rollers.

Try to wash your hair less often. The fewer times you wash your hair the better (but obviously you will have to find your own balance between reducing the frequency of washes and what you feel comfortable with).

Avoid shampoos and conditioners with lots of chemicals: try using a baby shampoo.

Avoid hair dyes and colourants, unless they are completely organic (plant-based), with no added chemicals.

Avoid perms.

If you have very long hair, then having it cut to a shorter style may help.

treatment; some drugs, or combinations of drugs, are more likely to cause mucositis than others (see Table 2.10). This oral mucositis usually comes on a few days after the drugs have been given and settles within about a week. The soreness can vary considerably in its severity. Often it is no more than a slight discomfort, but sometimes it can be very distressing, with the development of mucosal ulceration. Because the patient is often neutropenic as well, the soreness may be aggravated by the development of fungal infections in the mouth, most commonly oral monilia, which shows up as small whitish patches on the mucosa and the surface of the tongue. These infections are also common in people who are having steroids as part of their treatment. When mouth soreness develops it can also affect the sense of taste, so people often complain that things taste different, or that they cannot taste things so well whilst they are having their chemotherapy.

If a particular regimen is likely to cause mucositis then sucking crushed ice for 15–30 min before the cytotoxics are given, and continuing until about half an hour after the drugs have been administered, can sometimes prevent mouth soreness. One drug that is particularly associated with oral mucositis is methotrexate. The risk is usually dose-dependant and if higher doses of the drug are being used then this giving an iv dose of folinic acid (leucovorin) at the same time as the

TABLE 2.10 Cytotoxic drugs which commonly cause oral mucositis

Capecitabine	Hydroxyurea
Carboplatin	Lomustine
Chlorambucil	Melphalan
Cisplatin	Mercaptopurine
Cyclophosphamide	Methotrexate
Dacarbazine	Mitomycin
Dactinomycin,	Paclitaxel
Daunorubicin	Raltitrexed
Doxorubicin	Vinblastine
Etoposide	Vincristine
Fluorouracil	

methotrexate, and following this with a course of leucovorin tablets for a day or two can often prevent the problem (see page 28). If mucositis does develop after methotrexate administration, and folinic acid has not been given, then giving the tablets for a few days will often help. If someone does complain of a sore mouth after their chemotherapy then it is always important to check for the presence of oral monilia as this can readily be resolved with a course of an antifungal drug like nystatin, or amphotericin, for a few days. Oral soreness can also be eased by using a painkilling mouthwash such as Difflam Oral. Some people find using a full-strength mouthwash stings, and diluting it with an equal amount of warm water may help. An alternative is to suggest patients make their own mouthwash using soluble aspirin, dissolving a couple of tablets in a glass of warm water and using this to rinse their mouth well three or four times a day. If mouth ulcers develop, then there is a wide range of gels, pastes and sprays that may help these include Bonjela gel, Biora gel, Medijel, Rinstead contact pastilles.

More general advice for avoiding or easing oral mucositis includes ensuring that patients maintain good oral hygiene (see Table 2.11) and changing their diet to avoid foods and

TABLE 2.11 Advice for patients to reduce their risk of oral soreness

Have a routine check-up with your dentist before you start treatment, to make sure there are no obvious tooth or gum problems that need to be dealt with before your chemotherapy.

Maintain good oral hygiene; this means cleaning your teeth at least twice a day. Using a normal toothbrush can be uncomfortable, so using a soft toothbrush, or a child's brush, might help.

You may find that your usual toothpaste makes your mouth and gums sore, and changing to a brand for 'sensitive teeth', like Sensodyne Original or Macleans Sensitive, might help.

Mouthwashes can also be useful, and you can try these if you find that brushing your teeth is really painful. There are preparations you can get from your chemist or supermarket that help to prevent infection, these include chlorhexidine, Corsodyl, and thymol.

For simply keeping your mouth clean you can make your own mouthwash with a teaspoonful of baking powder (sodium bicarbonate) dissolved in a glass of warm water, and use this to rinse out your mouth thoroughly morning and night.

Keeping your mouth moist with regular fluids. You should be drinking at least 2 l of fluid every day during your treatment, but supplementing this with regular sips of water or other soft drinks can help (fizzy water, or fizzy drinks, tend to be better than still fluids).

Try to avoid, or reduce, smoking, alcohol and caffeine (in tea and coffee) all of which tend to make your mouth dry and can make soreness worse

drinks that may make their mouth sore if the mucosa is sensitive: these include very hot and spicy foods, vinegar, salt, neat spirits (whisky, brandy, gin, etc.) and acid drinks like grapefruit juice and some types of orange juice.

Suggestions for Further Reading

Mitchell EP. Gastrointestinal toxicity of antineoplastic agents. Semin Oncol. 2006;33:106–20.
Keefe DM, Schubert MM, Elting LS, et al. Updated clinical practice guidelines for the prevention and treatment of mucositis. Cancer. 2007;109:820–31.

Reduced Fertility

As with other side effects, the risk of any effect on fertility is related to which drugs are used, and the doses given, and the length of time the treatment goes on for. Some cytotoxic treatments carry a very high risk of infertility, whereas with others there is almost no risk. The drugs that are most frequently associated with infertility are the alkylating agents. So if fertility is an issue then choosing regimens that either avoid these drugs completely, or keep their doses to a minimum, whilst maintaining anti-cancer efficacy, should be the objective. For example, in Hodgkin lymphoma, where young people are frequently affected, the original MOPP regimen, containing the potent alkylating agent nitrogen mustard leading to almost universal sterility, has largely been supplanted by ABVD, where the risk of infertility appears to be minimal.

For men, cytotoxics can have a direct effect on spermatogenesis, with a reduction in the sperm count becoming apparent within 3 weeks of starting treatment. This risk relates almost entirely to which drugs are used (see Table 2.12). But in some types of cancer, in particular cancer of the testicle, a reduced level of fertility, with a lower than normal sperm count, may actually be part of the man's condition, even before they begin any treatment.

For women, cytotoxics may cause destruction of the ovarian follicles, resulting in failure of ovulation, amenorrhoea, and sterility. The drugs may also lead to a reduction in ovarian hormone production, leading to menopausal symptoms. The risk of loss of ovarian activity with cytotoxic treatment increases the closer a woman is to the natural menopause. Sometimes, especially in younger women, cytotoxic treatment leads only to a temporary loss of ovarian activity, so the periods stop during treatment, and for anywhere from 3 to 18 months afterwards, but then can start again. The risk of permanent ovarian suppression is confined to the alkylating agents, and is largely dose dependant. Other drugs may cause a temporary interruption in ovarian function.

For men, if there is a chance that treatment will affect their fertility, they should always be offered the chance of

TABLE 2.12 Chemotherapy and male fertility

Drugs likely to cause permanent or prolonged azoospermia

Busulfan	Ifosfamide
Carmustine	Lomustine
Chlorambucil	Melphalan
Cisplatin	Nitrogen mustard
Cyclophosphamide	Procarbazine
Dactinomycin	

Drugs which may cause some temporary reduction in sperm count when used alone, but can have an additive effect on fertility in combination regimens

Amsacrine	Fluorouracil
Bleomycin	Fludarabine
Carboplatin	Mercaptopurine
Cytaribine	Methotrexate
Dacarbazine	Mitoxantrone
Daunorubicin	Thioguanine
Doxorubicin	Thiotepa
Epirubicin	Vinblastine
Etoposide	Vincristine

Drugs with an unknown effect on spermatogenesis

Docetaxel	Oxaliplatin
Irinotecan	Paclitaxel
Monoclonal antibodies	Small molecule TK inhibitors

sperm banking before beginning therapy. Freezing the sample does further reduce the quality of the sperm, but once they are frozen they can be kept indefinitely without any further deterioration and this does offer some hope of fathering future children. For women, the options are more limited. Freezing and storage of embryos that can be thawed and reimplanted into the womb after treatment is possible, but delaying treatment long enough for this to be arranged will not usually be possible. Even with this technique the chances of a successful pregnancy are probably still only about one in five. An operation to take away eggs (oocytes) from the ovary and have these frozen, or taking away pieces of ovarian tissue for storage (that could be replaced after treatment to try and make the ovaries work again), are both possible, but are really experimental approaches that are still being developed, with, at the moment, very little chance of success. Another option is egg donation, where, after the treatment is over, the patient's womb could be implanted with eggs donated by another woman. This has resulted in successful pregnancies for some women after their ovaries have failed as a result of chemotherapy.

There are two other points to mention. Firstly, because of the unpredictability of the effects of cytotoxics on fertility, it would be wrong to think that having treatment acts as a reliable form of contraception. So if patients are practising birth control, they should be advised continue this while they having their chemotherapy.

Secondly, people can be reassured that studies have shown that if fertility is reduced, but returns after chemotherapy, or if it was unaffected by treatment, the drugs that they have had will not lead to any increase in the chances of birth defects in children that they may father, or give birth to, in the future.

Suggestions for Further Reading

Banks E, Reeves G. Pregnancy in women with a history of breast cancer. Br Med J. 2007;334:166–67.

Lee SJ, Schover LR, Partridge AH, et al. American Society of Clinical Oncology recommendations on fertility preservation in cancer patients. J Clin Oncol. 2006;24:2917–31.

Jeruss JS, Woodruff TK. Preservation of fertility in patients with cancer. N Engl J Med. 2009;360:902–11.

Second Cancers

A number of cytotoxic drugs have been linked to the development of second malignancies, most commonly leading to acute myeloid leukaemia (AML). This problem was first identified following treatment with alkylating agents, in particular the nitrogen mustards. The risk varies with different agents (melphalan being some ten times more potent a carcinogen than cyclophosphamide) and increases with the overall dose of the drug given. Typically the leukaemia is appears some 5–9 years after treatment and is proceeded by the development of a myelodysplastic syndrome. Early estimates suggested that the likelihood of developing AML after alkylating agent therapy was about 1.5% at 10 years, but with greater awareness of the hazard this figure has probably now reduced.

The assumption is that it is the direct effect of alkylating agents on DNA that leads to their leukemic potential and so other cytotoxics which interact directly with the DNA chain might be expected to pose similar risks. An increased incidence of AML has been identified following therapy with platinum compounds, and the topoisomerase inhibitors (etoposide and the anthracyclines: epirubicin, doxorubicin and mitoxantrone). Isolated cases have also been reported after taxane-based chemotherapy. Among these drugs the risk appears to be highest with mitoxantrone with up to 4% of patients being affected, with the others there is less than a 1% chance of AML developing. Once again the risk appears to be related to dose-intensity, but unlike the AML linked to alkylating agents the onset is earlier, at 2–4 years post-treatment and not associated with an initial myelodysplastic phase.

Suggestions for Further Reading

Le Deley M-C, Suzan F, Cutuli B, et al. Anthracyclines, mitoxantrone, radiotherapy, and granulocyte colony-stimulating factor: risk factors for leukemia and myelodysplastic syndrome after breast cancer. J Clin Oncol. 2007;25:292–300.

Praga C, Jonas B, Bliss J, et al. Risk of acute myeloid leukemia and myelodysplastic syndrome in trials of adjuvant epirubicin for early breast cancer: correlation with doses of epirubicin and cyclophosphamide. J Clin Oncol. 2005;23:4179–91.

Travis LB. The epidemiology of second primary cancers. Cancer Epidemiol Biomarkers. 2006;15:2020–6.

Specific Side Effects of Cytotoxic Treatment

There are a number of side effects of chemotherapy which, although important, and occasionally serious, are limited to just a handful of the more commonly used cytotoxic drugs.

Peripheral Neuropathy

The peripheral neuropathy caused by cytotoxic drugs is mainly sensory. The first symptom is tingling, or pins and needles, in the fingers or toes. This gradually spreads to the rest of the hands and feet, and, if nothing is done, will go on to affect the remainder of the limbs. As the condition progresses, numbness of the affected areas will develop, and this leads to some loss of co-ordination, making fine movements like undoing buttons, typing, or tying shoelaces, more difficult. Loss of reflexes in the ankle and wrist are relatively early physical signs but weakness of the arms and legs is a very uncommon, late, occurrence.

Peripheral neuropathy is a recognized complication of treatment with three groups of chemotherapy drugs: the Vinca alkaloids (which include vincristine, vinblastine, vindesine and vinorelbine), the platinum compounds (cisplatin, carboplatin, and oxaliplatin), and the taxanes (paclitaxel and docetaxel). Of the vinca alkaloids vincristine is the drug most likely to cause neuropathy, and it may also affect the autonomic nervous system leading to constipation and, very occasionally, intestinal obstruction. As well as causing a typical peripheral neuropathy, oxaliplatin is also linked to a specific syndrome where intense, often painful, tingling sensations occur in the fingers and toes a few hours after the drug is given, lasting from a few hours to a few days, the symptoms often being made worse by exposure to cold: up to 90% of people receiving oxaliplatin experience this problem.

Usually the peripheral neuropathy is dose related, and comes on gradually, after two or three doses of the drugs, sometimes appearing only after treatment is complete. Numerous drugs have been used to try and prevent the neurotoxicity developing, but the results have been mixed and no one agent has been sufficiently successful to enter routine practice. If early signs of neuropathy appear then reducing the dose of the offending drug, or stopping it completely will usually help ease the problem, but sometimes this is an unacceptable compromise of the treatment. The neuropathy resulting from both vinca alkaloids and taxanes is generally reversible, although it may take months after treatment is over to disappear completely. With platinum compounds the picture is more mixed with the changes sometimes being permanent, although usually with low to moderate doses of the drugs there will be a recovery eventually.

Suggestions for Further Reading

Hausher FH, Schilsky RL, Berghonr EJ, Liberman F. Diagnosis, management and evaluation of chemotherapy-induced peripheral neuropathy. Semin Oncol. 2006;33:15–49.

Windebank AJ, Grisold W. Chemotherapy-induced neuropathy. J Peripher Nerv Syst. 2008;13:27–46.

Cardiotoxicity

A number of cytotoxics carry the risk of cardiac damage, including the anthracyclines, fluorouracil and vinca alkaloids. Cardiotoxicity is also a side effect of the monoclonal antibody trastuzumab (see page 98).

Doxorubicin is the anthracycline most likely to cause cardiac toxicity. Transient arrhythmias may occur in the first few hours after administration of the drug. These are most likely in people with previously abnormal ECGs. The arrhythmias

usually do not require treatment, and are not a contraindica-
tion to further doses of the drug. Very rarely more serious,
life-threatening, ventricular arrhythmias have been reported.
The more significant risk with the drug is chronic cardiomyopathy. This is dose-related. Early studies suggested that less
than 1% of people who received a cumulative dose of
<550 mg/m^2 were affected, with the incidence increasing to
more than 30% with cumulative doses between 550 and
1,150 mg/m^2. With greater awareness of this problem, and
better means of monitoring it, particularly the measurement
of left ventricular ejection fraction (LVEF), it is now clear
that the incidence may be higher and cardiac damage can
occur even at relatively low doses. For these reasons many
clinicians have reduced the maximum cumulative dose of the
drug to 450–500 mg/m^2. The cardiomyopathy leads to congestive cardiac failure, which may not appear until some months,
or even years, after the last dose of the drug. The heart failure
can often be difficult to treat and carries quite a high mortality. Apart from dose, other predisposing factors include age
over 70, pre-existing heart disease, and a past history of radiotherapy to the mediastinum. Most dose-schedules for doxorubicin give total doses below the 500 mg/m^2 level. For those
people with risk factors that might leads to problems at lower
levels monitoring of their LVEF is advisable; a pre-treatment
value of 45% or a fall to this level during treatment, would
usually mean that the drug is contra-indicated or should be
stopped. Epirubicin has the potential to cause similar cardiac
problems to doxorubicin, but the cumulative dose at which
these are seen is significantly higher, at between 900 and
1,000 mg/m^2. Chronic cardiomyopathy may occur with other
anthracyclines, and once again is dose-related: with daunorubicin 1.5% of people will develop cardiomyopathy at a cumulative dose below 500 mg/m^2, whereas between 500–100 mg/
m^2 the figure rises to 12%, and for mitoxantrone the suggested maximum cumulative dose is 160 mg/m^2.

A number of suggestions have been made to reduce doxorubicin toxicity. There is limited evidence that the risk of
cardiac damage is reduced if the drug is given by prolonged

intravenous infusion, or on a once weekly basis at lower doses. Also a number of agents have been investigated as cardioprotective agents during doxorubicin therapy, the most widely evaluated being dexrazoxane, but their value remains to be established. The liposomal formulation of doxorubicin does not permeate the blood vessels of the myocardium, and is associated with only minimal cardiotoxicity.

A further problem with doxorubicin is that when given in combination with paclitaxel there is a high risk of cardiotoxicity. Studies have now shown that this relates to the scheduling of the drugs, as the paclitaxel infusion delays doxorubicin clearance and prolongs its plasma half-life. The risk of cardiac damage can be minimised by giving doxorubicin first, with a delay of at least 30 min before the paclitaxel infusion, and limiting the cumulative dose of doxorubicin during treatment to 360 mg/m^2. By contrast, combining doxorubicin with docetaxel is not associated with an increased risk of cardiac damage, nor is there any increased risk if either taxane is given with epirubicin.

Both fluorouracil and capecitabine may cause cardiotoxicity. The signs of this range from asymptomatic ECG changes to angina pectoris and myocardial infarction, which may be fatal. The mechanism for these changes remains uncertain, although coronary vasospasm has been suggested. With fluorouracil they are most likely to occur within 72 h of the first dose of the drug, and are commoner with higher doses given by continuous infusion. When symptoms occur about half the patients experience angina, about 25% infarction, 15% arrhythmias, and the remainder either acute pulmonary oedema, pericarditis or cardiac arrest. The development of cardiotoxicity means that the drug should be stopped, in trials where patients have been rechallenged with fluorouracil after signs of cardiac problems there have been significant numbers of cardiac deaths.

Suggestions for Further Reading

Kristeleit R, O'Brien M. Cardiotoxicity from cytotoxics in the 21st century. Br J Cardiol. 2009;16:60–2.

Ng R, Better N, Green MD. Anti-cancer agents and cardiotoxicity. Semin Oncol. 2006;33:2–14.

Senkus E, Jassem J. Cardiovascular effects of systemic cancer treatment. Cancer Treat Rev. 2010;37:300–11.

Renal Damage

Cisplatin is the cytotoxic drug most closely associated with nephrotoxicity. The degree of injury to the kidneys is dose-dependant, and cumulative, single doses below 50 mg/m^2 seldom causing problems. Higher doses lead to renal tubular injury which in turn may lead to electrolyte imbalance, especially low sodium and/or magnesium levels in the blood, as well as reduced creatinine clearance levels and ultimately renal failure. These changes persist for months, and often years, after treatment is over; for example, it has been estimated that 4 years after chemotherapy with cisplatin men treated for testicular cancer have, on average, a 15% reduction in their creatinine clearance.

As well as dose-limitation cisplatin nephrotoxicity can also be reduced by using a forced diuresis, with large volumes of intravenous normal saline before and after administration of the drug. This dilutes the concentration of cisplatin in the renal tubules and speeds its transit through the kidneys. Originally the schedules for the saline infusions lasted anywhere from 24 to 36 h, necessitating that treatment be given on an in-patient basis, but these have been modified over time and it is now often possible to give the treatment on a day-patient basis. A number of chemicals have been evaluated as possible agents to reduce the renal toxicity of cisplatin, the most widely tested being amifostine, but none of these has proved sufficiently successful to enter routine practice.

Carboplatin was developed as an analogue of cisplatin specifically to find a less nephrotoxic alternative. Carboplatin does cause less damage to the kidneys, only causing problems when given at high doses, but it does carry a greater risk of myelosuppression than cisplatin. To minimize the risk of renal damage carboplatin dosing is directly related to renal function (see page 46).

Table 2.13 Cytotoxic hepatotoxicity

Hepatotoxicity	Recognised side effect	Isolated reports
Hepatocellular toxicity	Cytarabine[a]	Chlorambucil
	Mercaptopurine	Gemcitabine
		Pentastatin
		Raltitrexed
Veno-occlusive disease	Busulfan[a]	Dacarbazine
	Carmustine[a]	Gemcitabine
	Cyclophosphamide	Mercaptopurine
	Cytarabine	Tioguanine
	Mitomycin	
Chronic fibrosis	Methotrexate	

[a]Following high-dose therapy

Other cytotoxics that have been linked to renal damage include mitomycin, methotrexate, and ifosfamide. Problems usually only occur with either prolonged cumulative administration, or higher than normal individual doses.

Suggestion for Further Reading

de Jonge MJA, Verweij J. Renal toxicities of chemotherapy. Semin Oncol. 2006;33:68–73.

Hepatotoxicity

Three types of liver damage have been linked to cytotoxic drugs: hepatocellular dysfunction, veno-occlusive disease and chronic fibrosis.

Hepatocellular dysfunction is characterised by an increase in the blood level of liver enzymes and bilirubin. It has most often been reported with high dose cytarabine therapy and mercaptopurine but it may occur occasionally as a result of a number of other drugs (see Table 2.13).

Veno-occlusive disease leads to blockage of small blood vessels in the liver which in turn causes hepatomegaly, ascites and oedema, and may progress to be fatal. It has been reported after high-dose therapy with a number of alkylating agents and also in isolated instances with a number of other cytotoxics.

Hepatic fibrosis is a complication of long-term low dose methotrexate administration. The drug is usually only given in this way in the treatment of a number of non-malignant conditions, such as rheumatoid arthritis.

Suggestion for Further Reading

Floyd J, Mirza I, Sachs B, Perry MC. Hepatotoxicity of chemotherapy. Semin Oncol. 2006;33:50–67.

Pulmonary Toxicity

Bleomycin is the cytotoxic most widely associated with lung damage, leading to chronic pulmonary fibrosis. Some estimates suggest as many as 1 in 10 people receiving the drug may be affected. Typically the changes appear 1–6 months after treatment. The pulmonary toxicity is dose-related and usually only appears when more than 400,000–500,000 units of the drug have been given (bleomycin dose-labelling varies in different parts of the world, and outside Europe this equates to 400–500 units). Other factors predisposing to drug-induced pulmonary fibrosis include older age, poor renal function (delaying excretion of the drug, allowing it to concentrate in the lungs), and radiotherapy to the chest. Much less commonly bleomycin may cause an early onset interstitial pneumonitis, which may also lead to long-term fibrosis in some cases; this is not dose-related and is similar to a hypersensitivity reaction.

Mitomycin can cause a range of pulmonary toxicities ranging from transient bronchospasm, which resolves spontaneously a few hours after the drug has been given, to acute interstitial pneumonitis, to chronic pneumonitis and pulmonary fibrosis. Other drugs where lung toxicity, predominantly pulmonary fibrosis, has occasionally been reported include busulphan (the first cytotoxic to be linked to lung damage), methotrexate, cyclophosphamide, the taxanes and the vinca alkaloids.

Suggestion for Further Reading

Meadors M, Floyd J, Perry MC. Pulmonary toxicity of chemotherapy. Semin Oncol. 2006;33:98–105.

Skin Damage

Cytotoxic drugs may affect the skin in a number of ways but the two most important are extravasation (leakage of the drug outside the vein at the injection site) and hand-foot syndrome.

When cytotoxic drugs are given through a drip into a peripheral vein, even when the drug is given carefully, by trained skilled nurses, small amounts of the drug may occasionally leak outside the vein, into the surrounding soft tissues. It has been estimated that some degree of extravasation may occur in up to 5% of patients undergoing intravenous chemotherapy. With many drugs, extravasation is not a problem, and, at most, will only cause some slight brief discomfort. With a few drugs, however, any leakage into the tissues around the vein can cause quite severe inflammation, with redness, swelling and soreness. This comes on almost immediately after the extravasation has occurred, and, depending on the drug and the amount that has leaked into the tissues, may take days, or even weeks, to resolve. Occasionally long-term induration or even skin necrosis can result. The drugs most likely to cause irritation and skin damage when they leak are the anthracyclines doxorubicin and epirubicin, the Vinca alkaloids vincristine, vinblastine, vindesine and vinorelbine and the taxane paclitaxel.

If extravasation occurs then the tube through which the drug is being infused should be disconnected, but the needle into the vein should remain in place. A syringe can then be connected to the needle and used to draw back any remaining drug. If the extravasation involves anthracyclines then ice packs should then be placed on the surrounding skin, and the arm kept elevated. For leakage of Vinca alkaloids or paclitaxel a warm compress should be applied. In addition specific antidotes have been recommended. For anthracycline extravasation topical application of dimethyl sulfoxide may help and more recently intravenous infusions of desrasoxane (Savene), started within 6 h of the leakage, have also been shown to be of value. Desresoxane helps prevent free radical formation which is an important component of anthracycline-related extravasation tissue necrosis. There is also some evidence that dimethyl sulphoxide (DMSO) may be beneficial, as well as being a free-radical scavenger this chemical increases tissue permeability which might help diffuse the extravasated drug. For Vinca alkaloid and paclitaxel leakage immediate local subcutaneous injection of hyaluronidase is beneficial. Hyaluronidase causes the release of fluid into the extracellular space which helps to dilute the extravasated drug. Using an anti-inflammatory, or antihistamine cream on the affected area for a week or so afterwards can also help. Very occasionally if chronic painful skin damage results hyperbaric oxygen therapy, or surgery, with removal of the affected soft tissues and skin grafting, may be necessary (Table 2.14).

In recent years cytotoxic extravasation has featured increasingly in legal claims by patients. So if it does occur it should not only be treated meticulously, but also all aspects of the incident should be carefully documented.

A completely different type of skin damage which can occur with a number of cytotoxic drugs including fluorouracil, capecitabine, irinotecan, the taxanes and cytarabine is hand-foot syndrome (also known as palmar-plantar erythrodysesthesia, or acral erythema). In hand-foot syndrome the skin on the palms of the hands and soles of the feet becomes red and sore, and may actually begin to blister and peel. Sometimes the pain from this can be so severe that narcotic analgesics are needed to control it. It usually only comes on gradually,

TABLE 2.14 Management of cytotoxic extravasation

Drug	Non-pharmacological	Pharmacological
Anthracyclines	Cold compress immediately for 20 min, then qds for 3 days	Desresoxane iv infusion within 6 h, repeat on days 2 and 3
		DMSO sc at extravasation site 3–4 times daily for 7–14 days
		Topical antihistamine or steroid
Vinca alkaloids, Taxanes	Warm compress immediately for 20 min, then qds for 3 days	Hyaluronidase sc at six sites around the area of extravasation
		Topical antihistamine or steroid

with higher doses of the drugs, and adjusting the dose will often ease the problem. Sometimes taking tablets of Vitamin B6 (pyridoxine) at a dose of 200 mg daily will give some symptomatic relief.

Suggestions for Further Reading

Cassagnol M, McBride A. Management of chemotherapy extravasations. US Pharm. 2009;3 (9 Oncol Suppl):3–11.
Goolsby TV, Lombardo FA. Extravasation of chemotherapeutic agents: prevention and treatment. Semin Oncol. 2006;33:139–43.
Schulmeister L. Preventing and managing vesicant chemotherapy extravasations. J Support Oncol. 2010;8:212–15.

Ototoxicity

Cisplatin damages the outer hair cells in the organ of Corti in the inner ear. This injury can lead to symptoms ranging from reversible tinnitus to irreversible hearing loss and vestibular toxicity. The risk of ototoxicity is dose and schedule dependant, being uncommon with doses of <60 mg/m^2/cycle. A number of drugs have been tried as agents to protect against cisplatin-induced ototoxicity, but none has so far proved successful. As a result dose-reduction is the only way of preventing severe, irreversible hearing loss.

Suggestion for Further Reading

Rademaker-Lakhai JM, Crul M, Zuur L, et al. Relationship between cisplatin administration and the development of ototoxicity. J Clin Oncol 2006;24:918–24.

Bladder Toxicity

The alkylating agents, ifosfamide and cyclophosphamide, when they are metabolized produce a number of chemicals which are excreted in the urine. A number of these are urotoxic, and can cause irritation to the urothelium, leading to haemorrhagic cystitis. This is usually only a problem with cyclophosphamide when the drug is given at high doses, but with ifosfamide it is a risk at standard doses of the drug. The main urotoxic chemical which is produced is acrolein and this can be neutralized by mercapto-ethanesulfonate (MESNA). MESNA is routinely given as an intravenous infusion at the same time as ifosfamide, and it binds with acrolein, and other metabolites, to form stable non-urotoxic compounds which are rapidly excreted. MESNA does not have any anticancer action in its own right, nor does it reduce the effectiveness of the alkylating agents.

Diarrhoea and Constipation

Diarrhoea is most likely to occur following the administration of either fluorouracil, capecitabine or irinotecan. Depending on the dose and schedule used this can be severe or even life-threatening, and patients should always be made aware of this risk. For mild to moderate diarrhoea (the passage of 4–6 stools daily) dietary advice combined with regular doses of loperamide and a good fluid intake to avoid dehydration, should suffice. If

TABLE 2.15 Factors complicating diarrhoea

Severe abdominal cramping

Grade II or greater nausea or vomiting

Reduced performance status

Fever

Sepsis

Neutropenia

Obvious rectal bleeding

Dehydration

the mild to moderate diarrhoea is accompanied by any complicating factors (see Table 2.15), or if the diarrhoea is more severe, with the passage of seven or more stools daily, then more aggressive management is indicated. This would normally involve admitting the patient for intravenous hydration, and subcutaneous or intravenous injections of the somatostatin analogue, octreotide, titrating the dose as necessary to bring the situation under control. Prophylactic antibiotics may also often be indicated.

Constipation is most commonly seen with vincristine therapy, and usually appears 3–4 days after the drug is given. It is due to the effects of vincristine on the autonomic nerves, and may often be accompanied by signs of peripheral neuropathy. It is more likely in elderly patients or those on higher doses of the drug. Usually it will respond to mild laxatives and stool softeners, but occasionally it can progress to a paralytic ileus. This will usually resolve with conservative management over 7–10 days.

Suggestions for Further Reading

Gibson R, Stringer A. Chemotherapy-induced diarrhea. Curr Opinion Supp Pall Care. 2009;3:31–5.

Gibson RJ, Keefe DMK. Cancer chemotherapy-induced diarrhea and constipation: mechanisms of damage and prevention strategies. Support Care Cancer. 2006;14:890–900.

TABLE 2.16 Cytotoxic drugs likely to cause hypersensitivity reactions

Drug	Incidence of reactions
Bleomycin	1%
Carboplatin	5%
Docetaxel	20% (4% severe)
Doxorubicin (liposomal)	10%
Etoposide iv	2%
Oxaliplatin	20% (3% severe)
Paclitaxel	40% (2% severe)
Cabazitaxel	<10%

Hypersensitivity Reactions

These are most likely to be seen with the taxanes (see Table 2.16). The reaction is apparent within moments of starting the infusion and may include blood pressure changes (hypotension or hypertension), breathlessness, severe anxiety, flushing, a diffuse erythema, angioedema, itching and chest pain. The reaction is caused by sensitivity to solutes necessary to get the active drugs into solution rather than by the drugs themselves. The risk of reactions can be reduced by premedication. For paclitaxel and cabazitaxel this involves giving the steroid dexamethasone, together with an antihistamine and an H2 antagonist, for docetaxel usually only dexamethasone is given. Giving dexamethasone prior to docetaxel administration also reduces the risk of another complication of the drug: fluid retention, which can lead to oedema, pleural or pericardial effusions or ascites. If a reaction does occur then the infusion should be stopped immediately, and changed to intravenous saline, intravenous hydrocortisone and antihistamine should be given, and oxygen administered. In severe cases adrenalin may be necessary. The symptoms will usually rapidly subside, and often the infusion can be restarted after 30 min without further problems.

Liposomal doxorubicin causes similar immediate reactions in about 10% of patients, although the episodes are usually less severe. They only occur with first infusions. For those patients who give a history of allergies premedication with a steroid and an antihistamine may be a wise precaution.

In contrast to the taxane hypersensitivity reactions those seen with oxaliplatin and carboplatin tend to occur only after a number of courses of the drug have been given, typically 6–8 cycles. A number of desensitization protocols have been reported which may prevent further reactions, but often the development of hypersensitivity necessitates stopping the drug completely.

Acute hypersensitivity reactions have been reported with many other cytotoxics but they only rarely occur.

Suggestions for Further Reading

de Lemos M. Acute reactions to chemotherapy agents. J Oncol Pharm Pract. 2006;12:127–9.

Markman M. Managing taxane toxicities. Support Care Cancer. 2003;11:144–7.

Weiss RB. Miscellaneous toxicities. In: DeVita VT, Hellman S, Rossenberg SA, editors. Cancer: principles and practice of oncology. 7th ed. Philadelphia: Lippincott, Williams & Wilkins; 2005. p. 2602–14.

Tumour Lysis Syndrome

This is usually only seen with bulky, highly chemosensitive tumours, or in leukaemias with high blast counts. When cytotoxics are first given in the treatment of these cancers they may cause massive tumour necrosis which can lead to acute biochemical disturbances including hyperuricaemia, hyperkalaemia, hyperphosphataemia and hypocalcaemia. These can lead to acidosis and acute renal failure. Patients whose serum uric acid level or lactic dehydrogenase level (LDH) is raised prior to treatment, or those with poor renal function, are particularly at risk. The key to management of this complication is prevention. Patients who are deemed to be at risk would usually be given oral allopurinol, to reduce their uric acid levels, prior to starting chemotherapy and continue this throughout their treatment. This, combined with ensuring a good fluid intake will usually be sufficient prophylaxis. If the syndrome does develop then giving allopurinol, if it has not already been given, intravenous hydration and urinary alkalinisation are the first line management. If allopurinol has already been given then rasburicase may be used as an alternative. This is a recombinant form of the enzyme urate oxidase, which converts poorly soluble uric acid to water-soluble metabolites. In severe cases with it may be necessary to consider renal dialysis.

Suggestion for Further Reading

Howard SC, Jones DP, Pui C-H. The tumor lysis syndrome. N Engl J Med. 2011;364:1844–54.

Side Effects of Hormonal Therapies

Menopausal Symptoms

Generally hormone therapies cause fewer, and less serious, side-effects than chemotherapy. Many women being treated for breast cancer have virtually no problems at all from their hormonal treatment. Having said this, for a small minority of women the therapy can be very upsetting. The most common problems are unpleasant menopausal side-effects. These include hot-flushes, drenching sweats, vaginal dryness and soreness, mood swings, and irritability, loss of concentration and difficulty in remembering things. These are most likely to occur with tamoxifen, or goserilin. In younger women taking tamoxifen about one third will find their periods stop (if this happens it is still possible for the woman to become pregnant and she should continue contraception), one third will find they become irregular, and one third will see no difference, but all may get menopausal symptoms, as may some women who are postmenopausal and are given the drug. Recognising and sympathetically managing this problem is important as research has shown that up to 50% of women with breast cancer stop taking their hormonal within 2 years of starting, although they should take it for a minimum of 5 years. A variety of things can be done to try and ease these symptoms, and because this is a very common and significant problem, often underestimated by health professionals, these will be described in more detail.

If the symptoms are due to tamoxifen then changing the way the drug is taken might make a difference: either altering the time of day that it is taken, or breaking the tablet in two and taking half in the morning and half at night. Tamoxifen is made by a number of different manufacturers, and although all their products contain the same active drug some women find that changing from one brand of tamoxifen to another does make a difference to their symptoms. If none of these help, then for women who are past their menopause, a change from tamoxifen to an aromatase inhibitor, like anastrazole, letrozole, or exemestane, might well help, and will not affect the efficacy of treatment.

Sometimes simple lifestyle changes make things easier. Regular exercise, losing weight, and avoiding certain foods, particularly spicy foods, and certain drinks, particularly alcohol, may help to reduce the problem. Complementary therapies may also make a difference. There are a number of preparations available from pharmacists and health food shops which contain plant oestrogens (phyto oestrogens), the active ingredients include red clover, soy, genistein and black cohosh. There has been anxiety that because these compounds are a form of oestrogen, they might increase the risk of breast cancer recurrence but there is no evidence that this is the case. Vitamin E supplements have also been shown to help in some studies. Evening primrose oil, and ginseng are other popular remedies, and many women feel they reduce the number and severity of hot flushes and sweats, although scientific evidence for this is scarce. Studies have shown, however, that both acupuncture and relaxation therapies can benefit some women.

Sometimes prescription drugs may improve the situation. Hormone replacement therapy (HRT) is the most obvious choice but its role is controversial. Certainly it is often very effective at relieving the symptoms, but its safety is in question. At least one large clinical trial showing that women who use HRT after a diagnosis of breast cancer have an increased risk of recurrence, but this risk only seems to affect women over 50. So up to that age HRT may be given but thereafter, unless symptoms are very severe and all else has failed, then HRT is not to be recommended.

There are a number of other prescription medicines that can be considered as alternatives to oestrogen-based HRT, but none is as effective. A point of interest is that in all the placebo-controlled clinical trials evaluating these drugs the placebos have eased symptoms in as many as 1 in 3 women. The options include:

- Progestins: these may help reduce hot flushes. Some concerns have been raised about their use in women with a history of breast cancer although there is no clinical evidence of an increased risk of recurrence as a result of these drugs being given.
- Tibolone: this drug has weak oestrogenic, progestogenic and androgenic effects and has been shown helpful in reducing hot flushes, improving vaginal dryness and may be better than HRT in improving sexual function. However, because of its oestrogenic properties it is not usually recommended for women with a history of breast cancer.
- Gabapentin: this comes closest to HRT in easing hot flushes, helping in about 50% of women. It is not contraindicated for women with a history of breast cancer but can causes side effects of drowsiness or dizziness in about 1 in 5 people, although these tend to ease after the first week of treatment.
- SSRIs and SNRIs: selective serotonin reuptake inhibitors or serotonin noradrenalin reuptake inhibitors which are normally used to treat depression can often be effective in easing hot flushes. The mechanism for their action is not clear but they are widely used. Side effects may include headache, nausea, dry mouth, anxiety/agitation, sleep disturbance or sexual dysfunction but they tend to be mild

and short-lived. Drugs used include fluoxetine, citalopram, paroxetine, sertraline, mirtazapine, venlafixine and desvenlafixine. Although they are safe for women who have had breast cancer fluoxetine and paroxetine should be avoided by women who are taking tamoxifen as they can interfere with its action.

- Clonidine: this has mild to moderate activity in reducing hot flushes and is not contraindicated for women with a history of breast cancer but it often causes side effects of a dry mouth and sleep disturbance (insomnia or drowsiness). Although usually used to treat hypertension there is no evidence that it affects blood pressure in the doses used for relief of menopausal symptoms.
- Androgen therapy: low testosterone levels may contribute to loss of libido and sexual problems in some post-menopausal women and if tests confirm androgen deficiency then testosterone supplements may be helpful but will only be appropriate for a small minority of women.
- Topical oestrogen: there are a range of preparations for local administration of vaginal oestrogen including creams, pessaries, vaginal tablets and oestradiol-releasing vaginal rings. These are effective in relieving vaginal dryness. Only small quantities of oestrogen are absorbed into the bloodstream from these preparations and they have generally been considered safe for women with a history of breast cancer although some clinicians do have concerns over their use in this situation.

Suggestions for Further Reading

Hershman DL, Kushi LH, Shao T, et al. Early discontinuation and nonadherence to adjuvant hormonal therapy in a cohort of 8769 early breast cancer patients. J Clin Oncol. 2010;28:4120–8.

Hickey M, Davis SR, Sturdee DW. Treatment of post-menopausal symptoms: what shall we do now? Lancet. 2005;366:409–21.

Morrow PK, Mattair DN, Hortobagyi GN. Hot flashes: review of pathophysiology and treatment modalities. Oncologist. 2011;16: 1658–64.

Pachman DR, Jones JM, Loprinzi CL. Management of menopause-associated vasomotor symptoms: current options, challenges and future directions. Int J Womens Health. 2010;2:123–35.

Endometrial Cancer

Long-term tamoxifen therapy is associated with a small but definite risk of developing cancer of the womb. Approximately 1 in 500 women taking tamoxifen for more than 2 years will develop endometrial cancer. This is because tamoxifen affects different oestrogen receptors differently, inhibiting those in breast cancer cells, but stimulating those in the endometrium, leading to endometrial hyperplasia, and ultimately endometrial cancer. For this reason postmenopausal women who are taking tamoxifen should always be warned to report any vaginal bleeding so that this can rapidly be investigated to exclude the possibility of cancer. Happily most endometrial cancers related to tamoxifen therapy have been detected at any early stage, and the cure rate has been high.

Thrombo-Embolic Disease

Another consequence of the oestrogenic properties of tamoxifen is an increased risk of venous thrombosis. The risk is quite small with less than 1% of women taking tamoxifen getting deep vein thromboses. It is, however, advisable that women with a history of venous thrombosis should have an alternative therapy, such as an aromatase inhibitor, if possible.

Osteoporosis

The reduction in oestrogen level that occurs after the menopause mean that older women are prone to develop osteoporosis. Use of aromatase inhibitors increases this risk. Exemestane is a steroidal aromatase inhibitor, in contrast to anastrazole and letrozole, and it has been suggested that it might be less likely to lead to a loss of bone mineral density. Whilst this is probably true there is still an increased risk of osteoporosis even with this drug. Osteoporosis increases the risk of bone fractures, and these appear to be about 50% more common in women on an aromatase inhibitor than those on tamoxifen (the adverse effect of aromatase inhibitors on bone mineral density is in contrast to tamoxifen, which has a mild oestrogenic action on the bones, and hence offers some protection against osteoporosis). Although there are no definite national guidelines in the UK it is generally recommended that women who are to receive aromatase inhibitors have a baseline bone densitometry, DXA, scan, of their hip and lumbar spine prior to starting treatment. Depending on the result of this they may simply need advice on lifestyle measures to reduce the risk of osteoporosis (such as stopping smoking, reducing alcohol consumption, taking regular exercise and eating a healthy diet), or be advised to take vitamin D and calcium supplements. For women at high risk then adding a bisphosphonate, such as alendronic acid or risedronate sodium, to their drug regimen may be indicated.

Suggestions for Further Reading

Lester J, Dodwell D, McLoskey E, Coleman R. The causes and treatment of bone loss associated with cancer of the breast. Cancer Treat Rev. 2005;31:115–42.

Shapiro CL. Aromatase inhibitors and bone loss: the risks in perspective. J Clin Oncol. 2005;23:4847–9.

Van Poznak C, Hannon RA, Mackey JR, et al. Prevention of aromatase inhibitor-induced bone loss using risedronate: the SABRE trial. J Clin Oncol. 2010;28:967–75.

Hormonal Therapies for Prostate Cancer

The gonaderilin analogues, goserilin and leuprorelin usually have relatively few side effects. The most important of these is the risk of tumour flare in metastatic disease, when the drugs may initially cause a surge in androgen production during the first 2 weeks of their administration, before inhibiting release of the male hormones. This can be avoided by giving an anti-androgen at the same time as the gonaderilin analogue. Other side effects which may occur include 'menopausal' hot flushes and sweats, loss of libido and impotence, and irreversible breast pain and swelling (gynaecomastia) in up to 70% of men. Tumour flare is not a risk with the newer pituitary inhibitor degarelix which causes an immediate reduction in testosterone levels.

The anti-androgens may also lead to gynaecomastia, breast pain and 'menopausal' hot flushes. Giving a low dose of radiotherapy to the nipple area before starting the drugs can often prevent the development of gynaecomastia, similarly giving tamoxifen may also prevent breast swelling and pain. Because they do not reduce circulating androgen levels the non-steroidal anti-androgens, bicalutamide and flutamide, do not usually reduce libido or cause problems with erectile function or osteoporosis, whereas these may happen with the steroidal preparation, cyproterone. In addition cyproterone carries the risk of hepatotoxicity. The other main systemic hormonal therapy for prostate cancer, stilboestrol, carries the risk of cardiovascular toxicity due to thromboembolic complications.

These are all relatively immediate and recognizable side-effects of androgen-deprivation therapy but there are longer-term more subtle but more serious potential problems. Continued androgen-deprivation leads to a reduction in bone mineral density and decreased insulin sensitivity along with raised cholesterol levels and an increase in body fat mass. These factors mean that those men undergoing long-term treatment have an increased risk of osteoporosis, bone fractures, diabetes and cardiac disease.

Suggestion for Further Reading

Taylor LG, Canfield SE, Xianglin LD. Review of major adverse effects of androgen-deprivation therapy in men with prostate cancer. Cancer. 2009;115:2388–99.

Side Effects of Targeted Therapies

By definition, targeted therapies specifically attack cancer cells, with little or no effect on normal tissues – in direct contrast to cytotoxic drugs, which have similar actions on normal and malignant cells. Consequently targeted therapies generally have fewer, and less severe, side effects than cytotoxic drugs. These are summarised in Table 2.17, but a few features do merit further explanation

Trastuzumab and Cardiotoxicity

Numerous clinical studies have now shown that trastuzumab can cause cardiotoxicity. This takes one of two forms: subclinical, in which there is a reduction in the left ventricular ejection factor (LVEF) and clinical, with the development of cardiac failure. Overall subclinical toxicity occurs in about 10% of people and cardiac failure in about 2%. A number of factors which increase the risk of this side effect appearing have now been identified and are listed in Table 2.18.

This has led to guidelines being developed to minimise the risk of cardiac problems and those developed by NICE are typical, recommending that cardiac function should be assessed prior to treatment and trastuzumab should not be given to women who have an LVEF of 55% or less, or who have any of the following:

- a history of congestive cardiac failure
- high-risk uncontrolled arrhythmias
- angina requiring medication
- clinically significant cardiac valvular disease
- evidence of transmural infarction on electrocardiograph (ECG)
- poorly controlled hypertension.

The LVEF should then monitored every 3 months during treatment and if it drops by 10% or more from baseline or to below 50% then trastuzumab treatment should be stopped.

TABLE 2.17 Summary of side effects of targeted therapies

	Alemtuzumab	Bevacizumab	Bortezomib	Cetuximab	Dasatinib	Erlotinib	Gefitinib	Imatinib
Infusion reactions	+			+				
Fever/flu like symptoms			+					
Skin rash	+			+		+	+	+
Cardiotoxicity								+
Hypertension		+						
Hypotension	+		+					
Haemorrhage								
Thrombosis		+						
Nausea			+		+	+		+
Diarrhoea	+		+			+		+
Constipation	+							
Fatigue			+			+		+
Alopecia								

(continued)

TABLE 2.17 (continued)

	Alemtuzumab	Bevacizumab	Bortezomib	Cetuximab	Dasatinib	Erlotinib	Gefitinib	Imatinib	Lapatinib	Nilotinib	Rituximab	Sorafinib	Sunitinib	Thalidomide	Trastuzumab
Neuropathy			+												
Muscle/joint pain	+		+		+			+							
Headache			+					+							
Myelosuppression			+		+										
Oedema					+			+							
Pleural effusion					+										
G-I perforation		+													
Infusion reactions							+				+				
Fever/flu-like symptoms						+					+				
Skin rash									+	+		+			
Hand foot syndrome												+	+		
Pruritis									+			+			
Cardiotoxicity															+

Hypertension

Hypotension

Thrombosis

Nausea

Diarrhoea

Constipation

Fatigue

Sedation

Cardiotoxicity

Neuropathy

Muscle/joint pain

Headache

Myelosuppression

Tumour pain

Raised
bilirubin

TABLE 2.18 Factors increasing the risk of trastuzumab cardiotoxicity

Definite factors
Concurrent taxane use
Concurrent anthracycline use
Past treatment with anthracyclines
Age over 60
LVEF <50% at prior to treatment
Possible factors
Past or present hypertension
Body mass index (BMI) >25

The mechanism of the side effect of trastuzumab has yet to be fully clarified but unlike the cardiotoxicity seen with anthracycline cytotoxics (page 78) it is not dose related and appears to be reversible once the drug is stopped.

Suggestions for Further Reading

Morris PG, Hudis CA. Trastuzumab-related cardiotoxicity following anthracycline-based adjuvant chemotherapy: how worried should we be? J Clin Oncol. 2010;28:3407–10.
NICE Technology Appraisal 107. Trastuzumab for the adjuvant treatment of early stage HER2-positive breast cancer. NICE 2006.

Infusion Reactions: Cytokine Release Syndrome

Infusion reactions are common with the monoclonal antibodies and most often appear as hypersensitivity reactions with symptoms such as chills, fever, and an urticarial rash. Occasionally a more serious reaction may develop: cytokine release syndrome. This is thought to be due to monoclonal antibodies stimulating white blood cells to release large amounts of cytokines with produce an acute systemic inflammatory reaction. The most prominent symptom is severe dyspnoea, often with bronchospasm. As with the hypersensitivity reactions chills, rigors, urticaria and angioedema are also frequently present but in contrast to those reactions cytokine release syndrome usually appears 1–2 h after the infusion has commenced, rather than in the first few minutes of an infusion. Cytokine release syndrome is also often accompanied by signs of tumour lysis syndrome (see page 90), with hyperuricaemia and hypercalcaemia. Cytokine release syndrome is a potentially fatal complication of treatment and requires emergency treatment. It is most likely in patients with a high tumour burden and those with pre-existing lung disease. If possible alternative treatments should be used for these patients. Cytokine release syndrome has most often been reported with rituximab and alemtuzumab but may rarely occur with other anti-cancer monoclonal antibodies.

Targeted Therapies and Skin Toxicity

About 80% of patients given cetuximab, and a majority receiving erlotinib and gefitinib, will develop an acneiform skin rash within the first week or two of treatment, for some this will be quite severe. Although labelled acneiform the rash is not true acne and routine acne medications, such as benzoyl peroxide, should be avoided. It can appear as either a pustular eruption, or a pustulo/papular or follicular rash. There is no universally agreed treatment but routine measures include the use of mild soaps and skin moisturisers, with topical or systemic antibiotics if there is evidence of secondary infection (which is quite common). For more troublesome macular rashes topical steroids may help and for pustular rashes topical clindamycin may be beneficial. The rash usually fades spontaneously after a few weeks, leaving the skin dry and liable to crack. An unusual feature of these rashes is that people who suffer a more severe reaction are more likely to gain a therapeutic response.

Suggestion for Further Reading

Potthoff K, Hofheinz R, Hassel JC, et al. Interdisciplinary management of EGFR-inhibitor-induced skin reactions: a German expert opinion. Ann Oncol. 2011;22:524–35.

Chapter 3
Chemotherapy in the Management of Cancer

Breast Cancer

Breast cancer is now the commonest cancer in Britain. Every year more than 48,000 women, and 300 men, will find they have breast cancer. Overall nearly one in nine women will develop the condition at some time during their lives. The risk of getting the disease increases with age: half of all breast cancers are first diagnosed in women over the age of 65, and a quarter are first diagnosed in women over the age of 75. Breast cancer is getting more common. The number of new cases each year in the UK has doubled over the last 40 years. Although this increase in the frequency of the disease is worrying, it is offset by the fact that the cure rate is rapidly improving. In the early 1990s only about half of all women who had breast cancer could expect to live 10 years or more, but now this figure has increased to more than seven out of ten, and is expected to improve further over the coming years.

Oncologists have debated whether this improvement is due to the introduction of breast screening, with the detection of cancers at an earlier, more curable, stage, or the increasing use of adjuvant chemotherapy. This is a controversial subject but increasingly the evidence is in favour of systemic adjuvant therapy as the major factor in the improving outcome for women with this disease. When considering the use of adjuvant chemotherapy in early breast cancer two key questions are: who should receive treatment, and what

T. Priestman, *Cancer Chemotherapy in Clinical Practice*,
DOI 10.1007/978-0-85729-727-3_3,
© Springer-Verlag London 2012

treatment should they receive? One way to answer these complex issues is to adopt an historical approach.

Following the publication of the results from the early adjuvant studies in the 1970s it was possible, by 1980, to make clear recommendations. In terms of patient selection those women who had axillary node involvement at the time of their initial surgery should be offered systemic adjuvant therapy, whereas this treatment was not necessary for those women whose cancers were node negative. When it came to choosing what drugs to use the evidence suggested that pre-menopausal women should receive cytotoxic drugs, most frequently with the classical combination of cyclophosphamide, methotrexate and fluorouracil (CMF), and postmenopausal women should be given hormonal therapy, with tamoxifen.

Over the last 25 years it has become apparent that tumour size, receptor status and the histological grade of the cancer, are important prognostic factors, as well as the presence or absence of positive axillary nodes. As a consequence selection criteria have been adjusted to allow for these additional variables. But there is no absolute consensus as to how these criteria should be applied to individual patients. Currently at least three systems are available to make this decision. These are personal experience, prognostic formulae, and a number of on-line tools. Personal experience relies on the judgement of individual specialists, or groups of experts in multidisciplinary teams, making decisions based on their knowledge and judgement. The prognostic formulae take the patient's details, put them into an equation, and produce a number indicating their risk of recurrent disease. The most widely used of these calculations is the Nottingham Prognostic Index, which is as follows:

Nottingham prognostic index
- Tumour size (cm $\times$ 0.2) + lymph node stage (1 = node negative, 2 = 1–3 metastatic nodes, 3 = 4+ metastatic nodes;) + histological grade (1 = good, 2 = moderate, 3 = poor).
- A prognostic index <3.4 = good prognosis, 3.4–5.4 = moderately good prognosis, >5.4 = poor prognosis.

Although many clinicians, particularly in the UK, rely on this method it still only produces a score for that patient's risk of relapse, and there is no universal agreement as to the cut-off level above which systemic therapy is indicated. So, interpreting the answer from the formula, in terms of determining the treatment for a particular patient, is still a matter of personal judgement by the oncologists involved. The on line tools offers an alternative approach. The model for these is 'Adjuvant on line': backed by a database from the National Cancer Institute in the USA this is an internet service, which allows oncologists to enter the details of their patient and then to select a variety of adjuvant treatment options. The programme will then produce probable 5 and 10-year survival figures based on each treatment choice. This allows doctors to see which treatment is likely to be most effective and to get an estimate of the magnitude of the benefit. This system also provides data which are readily understood by patients, and so allows women to enter into a meaningful discussion with their oncologist in making treatment decisions. A number of similar systems have been developed and in 2010 the NHS in the UK introduced its own system 'PREDICT' available at www.nhs.PREDICT.

When it comes to selecting which systemic therapy to use there have been a number of significant changes since the 1980s, including:

- the routine use of oestrogen receptor (ER) testing, and the realisation that only those women with ER+ cancers will benefit from hormone therapy
- the discovery of the aromatase inhibitors as an alternative to tamoxifen for post-menopausal women
- the discovery of a number of new cytotoxic drugs which build on the benefits of the original CMF regime
- the recognition that cytotoxic treatment is beneficial in post-menopausal women, and contributes to increased survival, although at a progressively diminishing level, up to the age of 70 and possibly beyond
- the discovery of HER2 receptors and the recognition that women whose cancers are HER2+ may benefit from the addition of drugs like trastuzumab to their treatment regimen.

The discovery that only those women who had ER+ cancers would benefit from endocrine therapy initially simplified treatment decisions, but the advent of the aromatase inhibitors has complicated the picture. Clinical trial data suggest that these drugs are marginally more effective than tamoxifen in preventing relapse, reducing the risk of recurrence at 5 years by 3–5%, although their impact on overall survival still remains uncertain. Similar trials have also raised questions about the scheduling of hormonal therapy: traditionally tamoxifen has been given for 5 years but studies have shown that relapse rates can be reduced if either tamoxifen is given for 2–3 years followed by an aromatase inhibitor for 3 years, or tamoxifen is given for 5 years followed by an aromatase inhibitor for a further 3 years. There are also issues around toxicity profile (a greater risk of menopausal symptoms, thromboembolic complications and endometrial hyperplasia and cancer, with tamoxifen, and osteoporosis, with aromatase inhibitors), and cost, with the aromatase inhibitors being significantly more expensive than tamoxifen. At the present time there is no consensus on the optimum way to use endocrine therapy in early breast cancer and decisions will vary from oncologist to oncologist, and patient to patient, but there is a growing feeling that for higher risk patients initial aromatase therapy is probably the treatment of choice whereas for those with less aggressive disease either sequential therapy or tamoxifen alone might be recommended.

Other points to mention in relation to endocrine therapy relate to premenopausal women, and the sequencing of treatment. The aromatase inhibitors only work in post-menopausal women, and although tamoxifen may be used in younger women its effect on ovarian function is variable and unpredictable. In the past when ovarian suppression was considered necessary the choice lay between surgical removal, oophorectomy, or radiotherapy, a radiation meno-pause. Nowadays, however, these have largely been sup-planted by the use of injections of gonaderilin analogues, which offer long-term, but reversible prevention of oestrogen formation. The use of gonaderilin analogues in the adjuvant treatment of young women with breast cancer is variable. Although there are good data from clinical trials suggesting that they are as effective as cytotoxic drugs they are seldom used as an alternative treatment. However, some oncologists will use them in addition to cytotoxics, particularly in women at high risk of relapse, but the value of this combined therapy has still to be established by clinical trials. In the past when an adjuvant treatment programme combined hormonal and cytotoxic therapy the two modalities were usually given concurrently, but clinical trials have now shown that this reduces the effectiveness of cytotoxic treatment, and the pattern nowadays is to give cytotoxic therapy first, followed by hormonal manipulation. (The theoretical basis for the adverse interaction between endocrine and cytotoxic therapy is that the former reduces the level of cell division in the cancer, putting cells in the resting, G_0, phase of the cell cycle, where they are more resistant to cytotoxic treatment). Incidentally, giving radiotherapy concurrently with cytotoxic treatment does not reduce its effectiveness, although side effects, such as tiredness, may be increased.

When it comes to the choice of cytotoxic drug regimens for adjuvant therapy in early breast cancer there has been a similar evolutionary process. Clinical trials during the 1990s showed that the benefits of classical CMF chemotherapy could be increased by adding an anthracycline drug, usually epirubicin, to the combination. More recently trials have shown that combining epirubicin with a taxane, most often docetaxel, further increases the chance of cure. However, these additional benefits to come at the cost of increased toxicity: for example one major study with the epirubicin-docetaxel combination reported that 25% of women who had the drugs developed neutropenic sepsis. This means that in general oncologists will try to individualise the choice of treatment regimen for their patients, reserving the more aggressive drug combinations for women who are at high risk of relapse, and who are younger and fitter, whilst less intensive schedules are appropriate for older, frailer and lower risk women. Although studies have shown that cytotoxic treatment may have a positive impact on survival in women up to the age of 70, the benefit diminishes steadily over the age of 50 and so its use in women over 60 is, once again, a matter of weighing up the risks and benefits for individual patients. Over 70 the benefits are less certain, and the risk of significant toxicity increases dramatically, so cytotoxic treatment is less often used and frequently focuses on gentler therapies such as oral capecitabine.

For those women who have HER2+ cancers the addition of trastuzumab to their drug regimen has been shown to further reduce the risk of relapse. However, the extent of this benefit has been exaggerated by the media with an overall reduction of the relapse rate by only a matter of 2% or 3%. There was initial uncertainty over the duration of treatment necessary, but most oncologists are now using a 1 year course of the drug following conventional cytotoxic therapy.

In 2005 those women who had breast cancers which were negative for oestrogen, progesterone and HER2 receptors became defined as having 'triple-negative breast cancer'. Triple-negative cancers typically behave more aggressively than other types of breast cancer but do appear to be more sensitive to cytotoxic therapy. An aggressive approach is usually adopted in adjuvant chemotherapy regimens for these tumours with a typical schedule being cyclophosphamide and epirubicin being followed by a taxane. The platinum drugs, cisplatin and carboplatin, which are not generally used in breast cancer treatment are active in these tumours as is the anti-angiogenic agent bevacizumab and these drugs may play a part in the adjuvant treatment of triple-negative cancers in the future.

When it comes to the treatment of relapsed, metastatic, breast cancer the choice of systemic therapy depends on whether the receptor status of the tumour, and whether there has been previous systemic adjuvant therapy. In the past it has always been assumed that the receptor status of metastases would be the same as the primary cancer but it is now apparent that in about 15% of patients this is not the case and so, if possible, a metastasis should be biopsied to recheck the presence or absence of receptors.

If the cancer is ER+ then hormonal therapy would usually be the first option, unless the disease appears particularly aggressive, when cytotoxics would be preferred. If an endocrine agent, such as tamoxifen or an aromatase inhibitor, has been given previously as adjuvant therapy, then if the disease-free interval to relapse has been more than a couple of years the same agent could be re-tested, for shorter intervals an alternative drug would usually be chosen.

Once the cancer is no longer be responsive to hormonal manipulation cytotoxics can be introduced. Unless the disease is particularly aggressive the recommendation is for single agent therapy in this situation with drugs such as docetaxel, vinborelbine or capecitabine, the latter being attractive as an oral option. For more aggressive disease then a combination of a taxane with either an anthracycline, gemcitabine or capecitabine are possible combinations, the choice of drugs being influenced in part by what treatment the woman has received previously.

For those women whose cancers are HER2+ there is new evidence that combining trastuzumab with another HER2+ receptor inhibitor, pertuzumab and the cytotoxic docetaxel, may increase the length of remission by 6 months or more compared to the two drug combination.

Suggestions for Further Reading

Amir E, Clemons M, Purdie CA, et al. Tissue confirmation of disease recurrence in breast cancer patients: pooled analysis of multicentre, multi-disciplinary prospective studies. Cancer Treat Rev. 2012:38 in press.

Baselga J, Cortes J, Kim S-B, et al. Pertuzumab plus trastuzumab plus docetaxel for metastatic breast cancer. N Engl J Med. 2012; 366:109–19.

Benson JR, Jatoi I, Keisch M, et al. Early breast cancer. Lancet. 2009;373:1463–79.

Coleman RE, Bertelli G, Beaumont T, et al. UK guidance document: treatment of metastatic breast cancer. Clin Oncol. 2012:24:169–76.

Dowsett M, Cuzick J, Ingle J. Meta-analysis of breast cancer outcomes in adjuvant trials of aromatase inhibitors versus tamoxifen. J Clin Oncol. 2010;28:509–18.

Early Breast Cancer Trialists Collaborative Group. Comparisons between different polychemotherapy regimens for early breast cancer: meta-analysis of long-term outcome among 100,000 women in 123 randomised trials. Lancet. 2012;379:432–44.

Foulkes WD, Smith IE, Rois-Filho JS. Triple negative breast cancer. N Engl J Med. 2010;363:1938–48.

McPherson K. Screening for breast cancer – balancing the debate. Br Med J. 2010;340:c3106.

Welch HG. Screening mammography – a long run for a short ride. N Engl J Med. 2010;363:1276–78.

Lung Cancer

Lung cancer is the second commonest cancer in Britain. Each year there are more than 35,000 new cases, with some 32,000 people annually dying of the disease. More than 95% of lung cancers are smoking related. Although the incidence in men is decreasing that in women is still rising, giving a current male:female ratio of 3:2. The average age at the time of diagnosis is 65, with less than 2% of people being under the age of 50. Lung cancer can be divided into two main types: small cell lung cancer, which makes up about 20% of cases, and non-small cell lung cancer, which includes adenocarcinomas squamous cell carcinomas, large cell carcinomas and poorly differentiated carcinomas, and accounts for the remaining 80%. The management of these two forms of lung cancer is quite different.

Small Cell Lung Cancer

Small cell lung cancer can be classified as either limited, if the disease is confined to the hemithorax of origin and the mediastinum, or extensive, if there is spread elsewhere; 60–70% of people have extensive disease at the time of diagnosis. Until the 1970s both stages of the disease were uniformly rapidly fatal, with survival times being measured in a matter of weeks to a few months. The advent of intermittent combination cytotoxic chemotherapy dramatically transformed the outlook, as these tumours proved remarkably chemosensitive with about 80% of people going into remission, and about 20% experiencing complete remissions. Unfortunately this good news is offset by two negatives: firstly, most people will relapse, and secondly, when relapse occurs second-line chemotherapy is of limited efficacy.

A wide range of drug combinations have been found to be active as first-line therapy in small cell lung cancer but the combination of etoposide and cisplatin (EC) has emerged as the most successful and is the treatment of choice.

For people with limited stage disease the best results are obtained when EC is given concurrently with radiotherapy to the primary tumour. However, this is quite an intense regimen and for patients who are less fit induction chemotherapy followed by radiotherapy is an option. Overall use of one of these schedules will lead to average survival times of 18–24 months with about 15–20% of people surviving 5 years or more, and possibly being cured. For people with extensive stage disease etoposide combined with either cisplatin or carboplatin is the usual treatment choice and this results in median survival times of 8–13 months.

When good remissions were first seen following chemotherapy in small cell lung cancer one problem was that more than 50% of people relapsed with brain metastases. This was because the drugs used had little or no ability to penetrate the blood brain barrier, so seedlings of tumour that had lodged in the brain were able to continue growing. As a result 'prophylactic' radiotherapy to the brain was introduced for people who went into remission, and this is still usually given today as it reduces the CNS relapse rate by almost 50%.

Although small cell lung cancer is highly chemosensitive initially once people relapse the disease is relatively resistant. Many will be too unwell for active treatment to be considered but for those that are fit enough the main options are either topotecan as a single agent or a combination of cyclophosphamide, doxorubicin and vincristine, which may lead to an increase in survival of 3–6 months.

Non-small Cell Lung Cancer

The cornerstone of treatment for localised disease is surgery, Although this has the potential for cure less than 10% of people are suitable for an operation, either because of the extent of their disease, their general fitness (many people will have severe respiratory or cardiac problems because of their chronic smoking), or their age. For some of these individuals, radical radiotherapy may be an alternative, but offers a lower chance of cure than surgery.

The following paragraphs describe the role of systemic treatment in non-small-cell lung cancer. This is one of the most rapidly evolving areas of cancer chemotherapy and there have been very significant developments in the last few years and further progress is likely over the next decade. However, a sobering comment on the world of cutting edge new technologies and state of the art clinical trial data was offered by a survey carried out by the Department of Health in the UK in 2010 which showed that only 51% of people with a diagnosis of lung cancer received any form of active treatment (National Lung Cancer Audit, 2010. Department of Health, London).

For many years there was uncertainty as to whether giving adjuvant chemotherapy after apparently successful surgery would improve the outcome, clinical trials over the last decade have given convincing evidence of a benefit. This is, however, dependant on the stage of the cancer: whilst the overall improvement in survival was about 5% following the addition of chemotherapy, in people with stage 1A tumours there was actually a negative effective whilst for those with stage II and III tumours the figure rose to 17%. The treatment was based on either cisplatin and vinorelbine or carboplatin and taxotere, given for four to six courses over 4–6 months. The benefit did not appear to depend on the histology of the cancer. Some studies have also looked at giving chemotherapy prior to surgery (neo-adjuvant treatment). Although this also appears beneficial there is no evidence that it is superior to post-operative treatment.

In people with advanced disease palliative radiotherapy has been the mainstay of treatment for many years. Although this can offer effective symptom control, with cough, dyspnoea, chest pain and haemoptysis being relieved in more than 60% of cases, often by just one or two out-patient treatments, there is no effect on overall survival. In the late 1990s an overview of previous trials showed that platinum-based chemotherapy could increase life-expectancy, albeit by only a modest 6–8 weeks. Since that time further trials have shown that a variety of regimens can extend median survival times to anywhere from 12 to 24+ months. But patient selection is a key issue. The chance of a benefit is strongly dependant on performance status, with fitter, younger people being the ones most likely to respond; histology and the presence or absence of genetic mutations are also major factors.

For fit patients first-line chemotherapy is based on cisplatin. For those with squamous cell cancers this drug is usually combined with gemcitabine whilst for those with other histologies the doublet is cisplatin/pemetrexed. These combinations can yield median survivals of about 12 months. For less fit patients substituting carboplatin for cisplatin or the use of single agent therapy with either docetaxel, gemcitabine, paclitaxel or vinorelbine are possible treatment options. Some people despite having advanced disease will initially be asymptomatic and it has been suggested that treatment may be delayed in this situation but the evidence from clinical trials is that even in people who are symptom-free the sooner treatment is started the greater the increase in life-expectancy.

Up to 50% of non-small cell lung cancers carry mutations of the epidermal growth factor receptor (EGFR). Positivity for this mutation is more likely in people who have never smoked and those who have adenocarcinomas. Clinical trials have now shown that for those whose cancers carry this mutation the EGFR tyrosine kinase inhibitors erlotinib and gefitinib offer better outcomes than conventional cytotoxic chemotherapy with median survival times in excess of 2 years. As a result routine testing for the presence of EGFR mutation in people being considered for chemotherapy is becoming increasingly widespread.

Another recent development has been the concept of introducing maintenance therapy for those who respond to their initial chemotherapy and there is evidence that in selected patients this may extend survival by a few months.

The improvements in first-line therapy that have been seen in recent years have encouraged increasing exploration of second-line treatment and there is evidence that some patients will benefit from this although the remission durations are usually limited to a few months. The treatment options are summarised in Table 3.1.

TABLE 3.1 Chemotherapy for advanced or metastatic non-small-cell lung cancer

Clinical scenario	Treatment regimen
First line therapy	
Fit patients (performance status 0–1)	
Squamous cell histology	Cisplatin + gemcitabine
Non-squamous cell histology	Cisplatin + pemetrexed
Adenocarcinoma with +ve EGFR mutation[a]	Gefitinib, erlotinib
Less fit patients (performance status 2)	
	Substitute carboplatin for cisplatin in the above regimens or use single agents (docetaxel, gemcitabine, paclitaxel or vinorelbine)
Maintenance therapy	
Non-squamous cell if did not have pemetrexed initially	Pemetrexed
Adenocarcinoma with +ve EGFR mutation[a]	Gefitinib, erlotinib
Second line therapy	
Non squamous cell	Pemetrexed, gefitinib or erlotinib
Squamous cell	Docetaxel, gefitinib or erlotinib

[a]Some authorities recommend gefitinib and erlotinib for all non-small-cell cancers exhibiting the EGFR mutation

Suggestions for Further Reading

Felip E, Gridelli C, Baas P, et al. Metastatic non-small-cell lung cancer: consensus on pathology and molecular tests, first-line, second-line and third line therapy. First ESMO consensus conference on lung cancer. Ann Oncol. 2011;22:1507–19.

Goldstraw P, Ball D, Jett JR, et al. Non-small-cell lung cancer. Lancet. 2011;378:1727–40.

NICE clinical guideline 121. Lung cancer: the diagnosis and treatment of lung cancer. NICE. 2011.

Shepherd FA. Maintenance therapy comes of age in non-small-cell lung cancer, but at what cost. J Clin Oncol. 2011;37:4068–70.

Van Meerbeeck JP, Fennell DA, De Ruysscher DKM. Small cell lung cancer. Lancet. 2011;378:1741–55.

Mesothelioma

Mesothelioma is a primary cancer of the pleura (>90% of cases) or peritoneum. It is almost always related to previous asbestos exposure, often 30–40 years previously. There are some 1,700 new cases each year in Britain, with a similar number of deaths. The incidence of mesothelioma is predicted to rise over the next few years to a peak between 2011 and 2015, with the number of cases rising to about 2,000 a year. Mesothelioma is commoner in men than women with a ratio of 6.5:1. The average age at diagnosis is 75. The overall 5 year survival is about 3%, with the median survival being about 9 months.

The very poor outcome for mesothelioma is in part due to the fact that it is usually only diagnosed at an advanced stage. For those few people where the disease is discovered sooner surgery, with an extrapleural pneumonectomy may be an option. For people with more advanced disease cytotoxic chemotherapy combining pemetrexed with cisplatin offers a chance of a response in about 40% of people with a median increase in survival of about 3 months, from 10 to 13 months, and this has become the treatment of choice in this condition.

Suggestions for Further Reading

Rena O. Extrapleural pneumonectomy. Br Med J. 2011;343:d5706.

Tsao A, Wistuba I, Roth J, Kindler HL. Malignant pleural mesothelioma. J Clin Oncol. 2009;27:2081–90.

Vogelzang NJ. Chemotherapy for malignant pleural mesothelioma. Lancet. 2008;371:1640–42.

Urological Cancer

Kidney Cancer

There are 6,000 new cases of kidney cancer each year in Britain, with just over 3,000 people annually dying of the disease. The average age at the time of diagnosis is 60. Renal cancer is twice as common in men than women. Smoking, obesity and hypertension all increase the risk of developing a renal cancer. Clear cell carcinomas account for more than 80% of renal cancers. It has long been recognised that a tiny minority of clear cell carcinomas of the kidney occur as a complication of the rare inherited syndrome von Hippel Lindau disease. The overall 5 year survival figure is 45%. This figure is improving, partly because an increasing number of renal cancers, currently about 30%, are diagnosed as incidental findings in people having abdominal CT scans for some other reason, and hence are discovered at an early, pre-symptomatic, stage.

Surgery, with either a total or partial nephrectomy, is the definitive treatment for renal cancers. Adjuvant chemotherapy has nothing to offer. Historically chemotherapy has had a very limited role in advanced renal cancer: cytotoxics have proved uniformly ineffective. The progestogen hormone Provera has been advocated but responses are rarely, if ever, seen. The cytokines interferon alpha and interleukin have been used but response rates are only of the order of 10%, with no good evidence of increased survival, and both drugs are associated with considerable toxicity.

The appearance of the newer targeted therapies has transformed this depressing picture. There are now a number of drugs which have been shown to have activity in this situation including sunitinib, sorafenib, pazapanib, bevacizumab, temsirolimus and everolimus. The effectiveness of these agents is at least in part explained by angiogenesis inhibition. The background to this is that in von Hippel Lindau disease (VHL) the VHL tumour suppressor gene is inactivated. This same abnormality has now been identified in more than 60% of sporadic clear cell renal carcinomas. VHL inactivation leads to an increase in levels of vascular endothelial growth factor (VEGF), platelet derived growth factor α (PDGFα), and transforming growth factor a (TDGFa), all of which stimulate new blood vessel formation, and hence support tumour growth. Sunitinib, sorafenib and pazopanib act primarily by inhibiting VEGF and PDGFα receptors whilst the mTOR inhibitors temsirolimus and everolimus acts at a later stage in the pathway by inhibiting signal transduction to the nucleus.

Clinical trials are still establishing the relative merits of these agents in advanced renal cancer but at the present time sunitinib and pazopanib appear the most effective agents offering an increase in survival times of 12 months or more but with so many drugs now available, and the prospect of more in the future, the outlook can only improve in this condition.

Suggestions for Further Reading

NICE technology appraisal guidance 215. Pazopanib for the first-line treatment of advanced renal cell carcinoma. NICE. 2011.

Powles T, Chowdhury S, Jones R, et al. Sunitinib and other targeted therapies for renal cell carcinoma. Br J Cancer. 2011;104:741–5.

Rini BI, Campbell SC, Escudier B. Renal cell carcinoma. Lancet. 2009;373:1119–32.

Schmidinger M, Bellmunt J. Plethora of agents, plethora of targets, plethora of side effects in metastatic renal carcinoma. Cancer Treat Rev. 2010;36:416–24.

Bladder Cancer

Bladder cancer is the fifth commonest cancer in Britain. There are about 14,000 new cases of bladder cancer each year, with 4,700 people annually dying of the disease. The average age at the time of diagnosis is 70. Bladder cancer is three times more common in men than women. Transitional cell carcinomas account for more than 90% of bladder cancers. The overall 5 year survival figure is 65%. This figure hides the fact that bladder cancer is made up of two different types of disease: superficial and invasive cancers.

Superficial bladder cancers are tumours confined to the mucosal lining of the bladder. They make up 70% of bladder cancers. Based on the microscopic appearance of the tumour cells they can be classified as low risk or high risk cancers. Low risk cancers, which account for 60% of superficial tumours, behave in a relatively benign way. High risk cancers carry the risk of transformation to invasive disease. Management of these growths is by an initial cystoscopic resection or diathermy of the cancer, followed immediately by instillation of a chemical into the bladder. The drug is introduced through a catheter at the time of operation, the catheter is then clamped for the next few hours allowing the drug to be partly absorbed by the bladder wall. For low risk tumours all that is then required is a regular follow up cystoscopy to check that there is no evidence of recurrence. For high risk tumours similar regular cystoscopies are offered but are usually followed by further drug instillations. For some patients with extensive high risk disease, where there is considered to be a very strong chance of invasive cancer developing, a radical cystectomy may be offered as an alternative.

The most widely used, and most effective, chemical for bladder instillations is bacille Calmette-Guerin (BCG), which was for many years used as a vaccine against tuberculosis. Quite why it is so effective in treating superficial bladder cancer remains uncertain. Solutions of a number of cytotoxic drugs may be used as an alternative to BCG, among these are mitomycin, epirubicin and doxorubicin.

For invasive cancers surgery is the cornerstone of treatment, with a radical cystectomy being offered. As bladder cancer is mainly a disease of older people many patients will not be fit enough for major surgery and radiotherapy is the treatment of choice for them.

Unfortunately 5 year survival rates are poor: about 35% after surgery, and 25% after radiotherapy. Giving adjuvant chemotherapy after surgery does not significantly improve these figures. However, a number of trials have used a variety of cisplatin-based regimens given pre-operatively (neoadjuvant therapy) and have shown an overall increase in survival of about 5% and this may be offered as a treatment option for fitter patients.

For people with advanced or metastatic bladder cancer the most widely used cytotoxic regimen for many years was M-VAC (methotrexate, vinblastine, doxorubicin and cisplatin). However, this was a toxic regimen and the combination of gemcitabine and cisplatin has now been shown to be as effective with far fewer side effects, and is the treatment of choice. It offers a response rate of about 40% and may increase survival by 4–6 months to a little over 12 months. For older, less fit people, for whom even this combination may be a challenge, single agent therapy with either paclitaxel, gemcitabine or pemetrexed can be given but response rates are only 10–20% and there is little evidence that survival is increased.

Although targeted therapies have been quite extensively explored in the management of advanced bladder cancer none has, as yet, shown significant therapeutic activity.

Suggestions for Further Reading

Gallagher DJ, Milowsky MI, Bajorin DF. Advanced bladder cancer: status of first-line chemotherapy and the search for active agents. Cancer. 2008;113:1284–93.

Kaufman DS, Shipley WU, Feldman AS. Bladder cancer. Lancet. 2009;374:239–49.

Shelley MD, Mason MD, Kynaston H. Intravesical therapy for superficial bladder cancer: a systematic review of trials and meta-analysis. Cancer Treat Rev. 2010;36:195–205.

Prostate Cancer

Prostate cancer is the fourth commonest cancer in Britain, and has recently overtaken lung cancer as the commonest cancer in men. There are more than 32,000 new cases of prostate cancer each year, with some 8,500 men annually dying of the disease. Between 1990 and 2002 the annual age adjusted incidence of prostate cancer nearly doubled in the UK. This was probably largely due to the availability of the prostate specific antigen (PSA) blood test, which allows the condition to be diagnosed at an early asymptomatic stage rather than a true increase in the frequency of prostate cancer. The average age at the time of diagnosis is 70–75. Increasing age is the greatest risk factor for developing prostate cancer, and it has been estimated that almost 100% of men in their 90s will have the disease. In younger men, in their 50s and 60s the disease tends to behave aggressively whereas in older men, in their 70s and 80s it is often indolent, progressing very slowly, causing few problems and needing little or no treatment. Prostate cancers are adenocarcinomas, and are graded according to their Gleason score, which ranges from 6 to 10, higher scores indicating more aggressive disease and a poorer prognosis. When prostate cancer spreads to other parts of the body it almost invariably goes to the bones. The overall 5-year survival rate is about 70%.

When considering its management prostate cancer can be divided into three stages:

- early disease: when the cancer is confined within the capsule of the prostate gland
- locally advanced disease: when the tumour has breached the capsule and spread into the surrounding tissues or pelvic lymph nodes
- advanced disease: when blood-borne spread to the bones has occurred.

Of those who present with symptomatic disease, as opposed to just a raised PSA level, about 50% of men will have early disease, 25% locally advanced disease, and 25% metastatic disease.

Options for the management of early prostate cancer include radical prostatectomy, radiotherapy (which may be either external beam – conformal or intensity modulated, IMRT, irradiation – or brachytherapy, with the insertion of radioactive seeds into the prostate gland), or policies of watchful waiting or active surveillance. To help decide which treatment is appropriate, men with early prostate cancer can be placed into one of three risk groups according to a number of parameters (Table 3.2).

TABLE 3.2 Risk stratification of early prostate cancer

	PSA		Gleason score		Clinical stage
Low risk	<10	&	<6	&	T1–T2a
Intermediate risk	10–20	or	7	or	T2b–T2c
High risk	>20	or	8–10	or	T3–T4

For those in the low risk group watchful waiting or active surveillance are usually recommended. Watchful waiting, which is usually more appropriate for older men (with a life expectancy of 10 years or less) who have few symptoms, is intended to delay treatment for as long as possible and to use hormonal therapy as and when therapeutic intervention is needed. Active surveillance is an option for younger men with low risk disease, or some with intermediate risk cancers but few symptoms. In this scenario the aim is to delay treatment for as long as possible but to use an aggressive intervention, with surgery or radiotherapy, as and when treatment is required. For men in the high risk group either surgery or radiotherapy is indicated and for those in the intermediate risk group the choice of treatment is less clear cut and is decided on an individual basis.

A key question is whether giving hormonal therapy in addition to surgery or radiotherapy can improve the outcome. Studies have now shown that there is a definite benefit from combining endocrine therapy with radiation, particularly in men in the high risk group. However, there is no evidence that hormone treatment improves the outcome after prostatectomy. The optimum timing of endocrine treatment (whether started before or after radiotherapy), and its duration (anywhere from 2 months to 2 years) remain to be confirmed. Therapy usually involves either a gonadorelin analogue (such as goserelin, leuprorelin or buserilin), or an anti-androgen (such as bicalutamide, or flutamide).

For locally advanced prostate cancer the options are either external beam radiotherapy (the extent of disease means brachytherapy is not appropriate), or endocrine therapy, or, more usually nowadays, a combination of the two.

Since the mid-1940s endocrine therapy has been the cornerstone of management of advanced prostate cancer. Nowadays the usual first-line approach is medical castration using one of the gonaderilin analogues and this will be effective in controlling the disease for the great majority of men, often for many months or even years. When relapse does occur the disease is termed castration-resistant prostate cancer (C-RPC). It is important to distinguish this from hormone refractory prostate cancer as C-RPC is usually still sensitive to other forms hormone therapy and so second line treatment with an anti-androgen, such a bicalutamide, flutamide or cyproterone, will often gain a further remission. Third and fourth line hormonal therapies are dexamethasone and stilboestrol. The place of the new inhibitor of androgen synthesis, abiraterone, has still to be established. One aspect of endocrine therapy in this context which remains controversial is total androgen blockade: this involves giving an anti-androgen along with a gonaderlin analogue as first-line treatment. Trials have shown that combining the two approaches to androgen inhibition does improve 5 year survival by about 5% but this benefit is relatively small and obtained at a cost of extra morbidity and expense which many oncologists feel is not justified by the modest improvement in outcome.

Traditionally hormone therapy has been given continuously for men with metastatic prostate cancer but recently it has been suggested that treatment might be equally, or even more, effective, if given on an intermittent basis. Clinical trials using various schedules have indicated that this might be the case, and even if there is no actual survival advantage then the time off-treatment has benefits in terms of quality of life for patients and the overall cost of treatment, so this approach is increasingly entering into routine practice.

Once the cancer does become hormone refractory cytotoxic treatment can be considered. Until a few years ago it was widely agreed that cytotoxic therapy played little or no part in the treatment of advanced prostate cancer. But in 2005 studies were published showing that giving docetaxel combined with prednisolone could actually lead to a median increase in survival of about 3 months. Although this is a modest benefit there is also evidence that giving cytotoxic

POSSIBLE ALGORITHM FOR THE SYSTEMIC TREATMENT OF METASTATIC PROSTATE CANCER

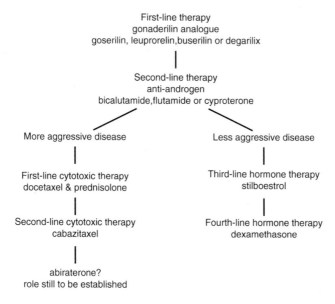

FIGURE 3.1 Possible algorithm for the systemic treatment of metastatic prostate cancer

therapy with docetaxel may help with symptom control and improve quality of life for many men. Recent trials have shown that on relapse the new cytotoxic cabazitaxel or the immunomodulator sipuleucel-T can offer a further increase in survival of a few months but at the present time the limited data on these compounds and their considerable cost are limiting their availability. These systemic therapeutic options are summarised in Fig. 3.1.

Finally for most men with bone metastases, who will make up the vast majority of this population, either a bisphosphonate or denosumab would usually form part of the treatment regimen, to help with control of pain and reduce the risk of one complications (see page 38).

Suggestions for Further Reading

Collins R, Trowman R, Norman G, et al. A systematic review of the effectiveness of docetaxel and mitoxantrone for the treatment of metastatic hormone-refractory prostate cancer. Br J Cancer. 2006; 95:457–62.

De Bono JS, Logothetis CJ, Molina A, et al. Abiraterone and increased survival in metastatic prostate cancer. N Engl J Med. 2011;364:1995–2005.

De Bono JS, Oudard S, Ozgroglo M, et al. Prednisone plus cabazitaxel or mitoxantrone for metastatic castration-resistant prostate cancer progressing after docetaxel treatment. Lancet. 2010;3761:1147–54.

Kantoff PW, Higano CS, Shone ND, et al. Sipuleucel-T immunotherapy for castration-resistant prostate cancer. N Engl J Med. 2010;363: 411–22.

Mottet M, Bellmont J, Bolla M, et al. EUA guidelines on prostate cancer: part II: treatment of advanced, relapsing and castration-resistant prostate cancer. Eur Urol. 2011;59:572–83.

Testicular Cancer

There are just over 2,000 new cases of testicular cancer each year in Britain. Although this is a relatively small number it is the commonest form of cancer in men under 45, with an average age of onset of 30. The incidence of testicular cancer has doubled in the last 40 years, and is still rising at 3–6% per annum. The reason for this increase is unknown. Germ-cell tumours make up more than 95% of testicular cancers and are made up of seminomas (55% of all cases) or non-seminomatous cancers. The latter is a heterogenous group comprising teratomas, embryonal carcinomas, yolk sac tumours and choriocarcinomas but the cancers are usually a mix of these histologies, often with a seminoma component as well, rather than being pure tumour types. Surgery, with removal of the affected testis is the first line of treatment. Testicular cancer has been a major success story for cytotoxic chemotherapy, 50 years ago metastatic disease was universally fatal, today, even for men with poor prognosis secondary disease, two out three can expect to be cured, and the overall cure rate for testicular cancer is in excess of 95%.

In the past radiotherapy to the para-aortic and ipsilateral iliac lymph nodes was offered as standard adjuvant therapy for men with early stage seminomas. Latterly trials have shown that low dose radiotherapy confined to the para-aortic nodes is adequate, and causes less long-term morbidity. Recently trials have also shown that a single course of the cytotoxic carboplatin is equivalent to irradiation. So currently the options for management are surveillance only, para-aortic radiotherapy or carboplatin. If the disease has spread to the iliac or para-aortic the irradiation plus carboplatin is recommended. For metastatic disease three courses of BEP cytotoxic chemotherapy (see below) is the standard of care.

The management of non-seminomatous cancers was transformed by the introduction of the BEP regimen in the 1970s. This comprises the three drugs bleomycin, etoposide and cisplatin. After an orchidectomy to remove the primary cancer 25–30% of men with early stage disease will relapse. Options for management after orchidectomy are close surveillance, with regular scans and measurements of tumour markers, offering treatment only when relapse is apparent, or a para-aortic lymph node dissection plus chemotherapy, or two courses of BEP chemotherapy. The choice is determined in part by the histological pattern of the tumour. For men who have metastatic disease the definitive treatment is four courses of BEP.

As present outcomes are so good the main focus for future development is the search for less toxic treatment regimens which will minimise the risk of long-term side-effects.

Suggestions for Further Reading

Feldman DR, Bosl GJ, Sheinfeld J, Motzer RJ. Medical treatment of advanced testicular cancer. JAMA. 2008;299:672–84.

Horwich A, et al. Testicular germ-cell cancer. Lancet. 2006;367:754–65.

Howard GCW, Nairn M. Management of adult testicular germ cell tumours: summary of updated SIGN guidance. Br Med J. 2011; 342:d2005.

Pliarchopoulou K, Pectasides D. First-line chemotherapy of non-seminomatous germ cell tumours (NSGCTs). Cancer Treat Rev. 2009;35:563–9.

Gastrointestinal Cancer

Oesophageal Cancer

Oesophageal cancer is the ninth commonest cancer in Britain. There are about 7,500 new cases of oesophageal cancer each year, with some 6,500 people dying annually of the disease. The average age at the time of diagnosis is 72. Cancers of the upper and middle third of the oesophagus are usually squamous carcinomas whereas those of the lower third are adenocarcinomas. Squamous cancers used to be the more common of the two, but in recent years the incidence of adenocarcinomas has been increasing and these now account for half of all oesophageal cancers. Overall cancer of the oesophagus is about twice as common in men than women, but adenocarcinomas are five times more common in men. The overall 5 year survival figure in the UK is 8%.

For people with localised squamous carcinomas of the upper third of the oesophagus chemoradiotherapy has largely taken over from surgery as the treatment of choice. The most widely used drug regimen in this situation is a combination of cisplatin and fluorouracil. For localised squamous carcinomas of the middle and lower third either chemoradiotherapy alone or chemoradiotherapy followed by surgery are treatment options, the latter probably offering an increased chance of cure but demanding a high level of fitness in potential patients. For localised adenocarcinomas of the middle and lower third of the oesophagus pre-operative (neoadjuvant) chemotherapy with cisplatin and fluorouracil is recommended. For adenocarcinomas of the gastro-oesophageal junction peri-operative chemotherapy is the optimum approach, giving epirubicin and cisplatin with either fluorouracil or capecitabine both prior to, and for a number of weeks after, surgery.

For patients with advanced disease chemotherapy has been shown to increase survival. There is no consensus on the optimum regimen but for both squamous and adenocarcinomas epirubicin, cisplatin and fluorouracil, or epirubicin and oxaliplatin with either fluorouracil or capecitabine are options and offer median survivals of about 9–10 months. For those with gastro-oesophageal adenocarcinomas which are positive for over-expression of HER2 receptors adding trastuzumab to cytotoxic treatment increases median survival by a further 2–3 months.

Despite the encouraging improvements in outcome with the greater use of chemotherapy in recent years it must be remembered that many of these figures come from clinical trials, which have included younger fitter patients. Unfortunately many people with oesophageal cancer are still too old and frail when their diagnosis is made to allow anything more than good supportive care, to maximise their quality of life in their terminal illness.

Suggestions for Further Reading

Allum WH, Blazeby J, Griffin SM, et al. Guidelines for the management of oesophageal and gastric cancer. Gut. 2011;60:1449–72.

Mariette C, Piessen G, Briez N, et al. Oesophagogastric junction adenocarcinomas: which therapeutic approach? Lancet Oncol. 2011;12:296–305.

Stomach Cancer

There are about 8,500 new cases of stomach cancer each year in Britain, making it the seventh commonest cancer. Unlike many other cancers, the overall incidence of gastric cancer is decreasing, the numbers in the UK having halved over the last 30 years. However, cancers affecting the proximal part of the stomach, the cardia, are increasing in frequency and now comprise the commonest form of stomach cancer. Some 5,500 people die annually of the disease. The average age at the time of diagnosis is in the early 60s. Cancer of the stomach is commoner in men than women with a ratio of 5:3. The overall 5 year survival figure in the UK is 15%.

Surgery is the cornerstone of treatment for gastric cancer but unfortunately only a minority of patients have operable disease at the time of their presentation. Studies of post-operative adjuvant chemotherapy have been done over the last 25 years but there is no convincing evidence of a benefit. However, trials using peri-operative chemotherapy, giving cytotoxic treatment both before and after surgery, have shown modest improvements in survival and this has now become the standard of care for people with operable gastric cancer in Britain and Europe, with epirubicin and cisplatin combined with either fluorouracil or capecitabine being the treatments of choice. In the United States postoperative adjuvant therapy with chemoradiation, using fluorouracil and leucovorin as the cytotoxic treatment is a more popular approach.

In advanced disease the cisplatin, epirubicin and fluorouracil or capecitabine regimens have been the most widely used and produce responses in up to 60% of patients with an increase in survival of 4–6 months. About 20% of gastric cancers overexpress HER2 receptors and studies have looked at adding trastuzumab to cytotoxic chemotherapy for these patients and have reported modest improvements in overall survival of about 2 months on average.

Suggestions for Further Reading

Allum WH, Blazeby J, Griffin SM, et al. Guidelines for the management of oesophageal and gastric cancer. Gut. 2011;60:1449–72.

Hartgrink HH, Jansen EPM, van Grieken NCT, van de Velde CJH. Gastric cancer. Lancet. 2009;374:477–90.

Okines AFC, Cunningham D. Trastuzumab in advanced gastric cancer. Eur J Cancer. 2010;46:1949–59.

Carcinoma of the Pancreas

There are about 7,000 new cases of pancreatic cancer each year in Britain, making it the tenth commonest cancer. About 6,400 people die annually from the disease. The average age at the time of diagnosis is in the early 70s. Cancer of the pancreas is equally common in both sexes. The overall 5 year survival figure in the UK is 2% and most people survive less than 6 months.

Surgical resection offers the only hope of cure but less than one in ten patients will have operable disease and even then the 5 years survival rate is only of the order of 10%. Clinical trials have looked at both adjuvant chemotherapy and adjuvant chemoradiation to try and improve these figures. The chemotherapy regimens have been based on fluorouracil or gemcitabine. Adjuvant chemotherapy seems to be of some value, possibly increasing 5 year survival from about 10% to about 20%, but chemoradiation remains controversial with trial results being variable: it is not widely used in Europe but is often given in the USA.

Many people with advanced pancreatic cancer will be too ill, and will deteriorate too rapidly, for chemotherapy to be considered. For those patients who are considered for treatment gemcitabine is the most active single agent. Over the last decade clinical trials have explored combining gemcitabine with a number of other cytotoxics including fluorouracil, capecitabine, cisplatin, oxaliplatin or irinotecan. Meta-analyses suggest that combining gemcitabine with a platinum drug or a fluoropyrimidine (fluorouracil or capecitabine) does increase median survival and one recent study has shown that a triple drug regimen of fluorouracil, irinotecan and oxaliplatin gave a median survival of almost 11 months compared to 6 months with gemcitabine.

Suggestions for Further Reading

Conroy T, Desseigne F, Ychou M, et al. FOLFIRINOX versus gemcitabine for metastatic pancreatic cancer. N Engl J Med. 2011;364: 1817–25.

Pliarchopoulu K, Pectides D. Pancreatic cancer: current and future treatment strategies. Cancer Treat Rev. 2009;35:431–6.

Vincent A, Herman J, Schulick R, et al. Pancreatic cancer. Lancet. 2011;378:607–20.

Colorectal Cancer

Colorectal cancer is the third commonest cancer in Britain. There are more than 34,000 new cases of colorectal cancer each year, with 17,000 people annually dying of the disease. There are about 22,000 new case of colon cancer and about 12,000 of rectal cancer each year. The average age at the time of diagnosis is 70. Colon cancer is equally common in men and women but rectal cancer occurs more often in men with a male:female ratio of 3:2. Most colorectal cancers are thought to arise from preexisting polyps in the wall of the bowel and about 5% are due to the inherited conditions familial polyposis coli or hereditary non-polyposis coli (these account for most of the cases in younger age groups). Wherever possible, surgery is the cornerstone of treatment. The overall 5 year survival figure in the UK for both colonic and rectal cancer is 50%.

In the 1950s fluorouracil was identified as the only cytotoxic drug to have any significant activity in colorectal cancer, but even so response rates were disappointing with only about one in ten people with advanced disease seeing a benefit. In the 1970s the addition of folinic acid (leucovorin), which prolongs the inhibition of fluorouracil's target enzyme, thymidylate synthase, brought about an improvement with response rates in metastatic disease rising to about 30%. Over the next decade a lot of work went into exploring different schedules of administration of the two drugs to maximise their efficacy. Regimens which evolved included low dose folinic acid and bolus injections of fluorouracil (Mayo), high dose folinic acid, bolus and infusion of fluorouracil (de Gramont) and prolonged intravenous infusion of fluorouracil (Lokich). During this time clinical trials also showed that the drugs had some activity as adjuvant therapy in earlier stages of the disease. In the mid 1990s three further active cytotoxics were introduced: irinotecan, oxaliplatin and the oral drug capecitabine, which is similar to fluorouracil in its mode of action. More recently a number of monoclonal antibodies have also shown some promise in the treatment of bowel cancer, these include the anti-angiogenic agent bevacizumab and the EGFR inhibitors cetuximab and panitumumab. With so many recent developments the role of chemotherapy in colorectal cancer is still evolving, and the optimum management is for patients to go into clinical trials whenever possible.

In stage III colon cancer, when the disease has reached local lymph nodes but there is no obvious distant spread, adjuvant chemotherapy is generally recommended for patients under the age of 70 (although often given, the value of adjuvant chemotherapy in people over 70 is uncertain and controversial with some major studies showing no increase in survival but an increase in treatment-related morbidity). With fluorouracil, leucovorin-based regimens an increase in 5 year survival of about 10% can be expected. Newer regimens adding oxaliplatin or the combination of oxaliplatin and capecitabine to these drugs, suggest this figure may be increase by a further 4% in patients under the age of 70.

For people with stage II colon cancer the benefit of adjuvant chemotherapy is less certain, with perhaps a 3–5% improvement in 5 year survival, and guidelines suggest it should be reserved for those people who are considered to be at high risk of recurrence. But some oncologists do question the value of this treatment, pointing out that of every 100 patients given adjuvant chemotherapy only between 3 and 5 will benefit: about 70% will have been cured by surgery and a further 25% will relapse despite having adjuvant drug treatment.

Incidentally, the 'Adjuvant on line' service (see page 107) is also programmed for colorectal cancer, to help clinicians, and patients decide on the whether treatment is appropriate, and which agents should be given.

In stage II and III rectal cancer the focus has been on combining chemotherapy and radiation. Post-operative chemoradiation, using fluorouracil and leucovorin, has been shown to reduce local recurrence rates and improve long-term survival. With the introduction of routine MRI scanning to accurately stage tumours pre-operatively it has been possible to clearly identify those cancers which are locally advanced and for these pre-operative chemoradiation is increasingly being offered. This neo-adjuvant therapy can lead to a complete response rate of about 20%, with no trace of the tumour being detectable at surgery. The initial trials looking at this approach to treatment used infusions of fluorouracil concurrently with radiotherapy and the hope had been that using newer agents like oxaliplatin or capecitabine might improve on these results but so far, disappointingly, this has failed to be the case, with the newer drugs increasing toxicity without increasing benefit. Incidentally, toxicity is often considerable with the combination of radiation and chemotherapy and this is s treatment that is only suitable for younger, fitter people.

In metastatic colorectal cancer the optimum management has still to be defined. Most bowel cancers spread to the liver, and when the disease is localised within the liver surgical resection of metastases may result in a cure. The criteria for considering surgery are widening all the time but at present about 15% of people with liver secondaries are eligible for surgery and of these about 30–35% will survive 5 years or more. Increasingly chemotherapy is being used pre-operatively to shrink the size and number of liver secondaries which further increases the number of people for whom resection is possible, and improves the outcome.

For people with metastatic disease for whom there is no possibility of hepatic resection survival averages 9–10 months. Giving fluorouracil-leucovorin chemotherapy increases this to an average of 12 months. Early studies adding oxaliplatin (the FOLFOX regimen) showed life expectancy extended to a median of about 15 months but later studies, using modified drug does and scheduling are reporting average survivals of 20 months or more. The use of irinotecan with fluorouracil (FOLFIRI) or capecitabine can give similar results. Adding targeted therapy, with one of the monoclonal antibodies, has the potential for further benefit.

The EGFR inhibitors cetuximab and panitumumab are only effective in people whose cancers do not have a specific KRAS mutation (these wild type KRAS tumours account for about 60% of colon cancers, so the majority of patients will be eligible for treatment), whereas the anti-angiogenic agent bevacizumab is not dependant on specific gene profiles. Adding cetuximab to the combination of fluorouracil or capecitabine and irinotecan increases overall survival in metastatic disease by about 3 months, although combining cetuximab with oxaliplatin and fluorouracil appears less effective. Adding bevacizumab to either oxaliplatin or irinotecan and fluorouracil or

**POSSIBLE ALGORITHM FOR TREATMENT
OF METASTATIC COLORECTAL CANCER**

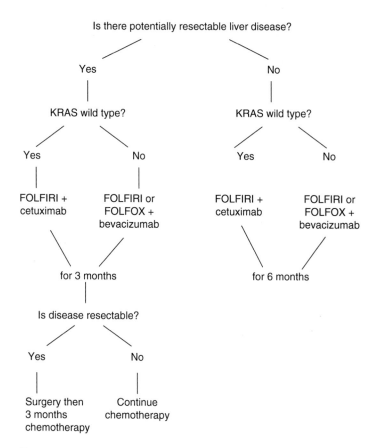

FIGURE 3.2 Possible algorithm for treatment of metastatic colorectal cancer

capecitabine gives a similar survival benefit (although in England at the present time NICE has not approved bevacizumab in this indication on cost grounds). These systemic therapeutic options are summarised in Fig. 3.2.

Suggestions for Further Reading

Andre T, Boni C, Navarro M, et al. Improved overall survival with oxaliplatin, fluorouracil, and leucovorin as adjuvant treatments in stage II or III colon cancer in the MOSAIC trial. J Clin Oncol. 2009;27:3109–16.

Cunningham D, Atkin W, Lenz H-J, et al. Colorectal cancer. Lancet. 2010;375:1030–47.

Grothey A. Adjuvant chemotherapy in colon cancer – is it worth it ? Eur J Cancer. 2010;46:1768–9.

Haller DG, Tabemero J, Maroun J, et al. Capecitabine plus oxaliplatin compared with fluorouracil and folinic acid as adjuvant therapy for stage III colon cancer. J Clin Oncol. 2011;29:1465–71.

Hewish M, Cunnigham D. First-line treatment of advanced colorectal cancer. Lancet. 2011;377:2060–2.

Primrose JN. Surgery for colorectal liver metastases. Br J Cancer. 2010;102:1313–8.

Weiser M. Rectal cancer trials: no movement. J Clin Oncol. 2011; 29:2746–8.

Gynecological Cancer

Cancer of the Ovary

There are about 7,000 new cases of ovarian cancer each year in Britain, with nearly 4,500 women dying annually of the disease. It is the fourth commonest cancer in women. The average age at the time of diagnosis is 70. There are many different histological types of cancer of the ovary but the great majority are adenocarcinomas, arising from the serosal surface of the organ; this summary focuses on these tumours. The overall 5 year survival figure in the UK is about 35%.

The first line of treatment for ovarian cancer is surgery, with removal of both ovaries, the fallopian tubes and uterus. Even when the growth has spread into the peritoneal cavity surgery is still recommended, with as much of the metastatic disease as possible being removed (debulking surgery). For those women with very early disease, where the tumour is well differentiated and confined to one ovary, no further treatment is indicated but for all others the standard of care is adjuvant cytotoxic chemotherapy. For women with poorly differentiated cancer confined to one ovary this may be carboplatin as a single agent but for all others it should be six courses of a platinum and taxane based combination.

Another approach to post-surgical chemotherapy is the addition of intraperitoneal drug administration, via a catheter through the abdominal wall, into the peritoneal cavity. A number of regimens have been used. One of the most recent, and most successful, involved giving conventional courses of intravenous cisplatin and paclitaxel, followed by intraperitoneal cisplatin 2 and 8 days later. Whilst this did lead to a prolongation of overall survival, compared to intravenous chemotherapy alone, it did cause a considerable increase in toxicity. At present intraperitoneal chemotherapy remains an essentially experimental treatment for ovarian cancer.

Ovarian cancer is chemosensitive and even with advanced disease about 75% of women will gain a remission. However, after about 18–24 months most will relapse with recurrent disease. At this stage treatment depends on their response to first-line chemotherapy, which falls into four categories:

- platinum-sensitive disease: this is a cancer that responds to first-line platinum based chemotherapy and relapses more than 12 months after completion of that therapy.
- partially platinum-sensitive disease: this is a cancer that initially responds to platinum based chemotherapy but relapses between 6 and 12 months after treatment has been completed.
- platinum-resistant disease; this is where the cancer responds initially but relapses within 6 months of completing platinum based chemotherapy.
- platinum-refractory disease: this where the cancer does not respond at all to platinum based chemotherapy.

For women with platinum-sensitive, or partially platinum-sensitive, disease then a further trial of either cisplatin or carboplatin, combined with paclitaxel, is recommended. For women with platinum-resistant, or platinum-refractory, disease single agent paclitaxel can be tried.

An alternative second-line (or subsequent) treatment for partially platinum-sensitive, platinum-resistant or platinum-refractory disease is the liposomal form of doxorubicin: pegylated liposomal doxorubicin. Another option for the latter two groups is single agent topotecan therapy.

Investigation of the newer targeted therapies has focused on bevacizumab and recent clinical trials have shown that when added to conventional carboplatin/paclitaxel-based cytotoxic chemotherapy for women with advanced ovarian cancer disease-free survival is increased by an average of 2–4 months. To what extent this will translate into an increase in overall survival is uncertain at present and cost considerations may also restrict the use of this approach to treatment.

Suggestions for Further Reading

Burger RA, Brady MF, Bookman MA, et al. Incorporation of bevacizumab in the primary treatment of ovarian cancer. N Engl J Med. 2011;365:2473–83.

Hennessy BT, Coleman RL, Markman M. Ovarian cancer. Lancet. 2009;374:1371–82.

Krasner C, Duska L. Management of women with newly diagnosed ovarian cancer. Semin Oncol. 2009;36:91–105.

Martin LP, Schilder RJ. Management of recurrent ovarian carcinoma: current status and future directions. Semin Oncol. 2009;36:112–25.

Perrren TJ, Swart AM, Pfisterer J, et al. A phase 3 trial of bevacizumab in ovarian cancer. N Engl J Med. 2011;365:2482–96.

Redman C, Duffy S, Bornham N, et al. Recognition and initial management of ovarian cancer: summary of NICE guidance. Br Med J. 2011;342:d2073.

Cervical Cancer

There are about 3,100 new cases of invasive cervical cancer each year in Britain, with 1,200 women dying annually of the disease. It is the seventh commonest cancer in women. The disease can appear any time after the age of 20 and there are two peaks of incidence at about 40 and in the early 70s. Seventy percent of cervical cancers are squamous carcinomas, 15% are adenocarcinomas and the remainder are mixed tumours. The overall 5 year survival figure in the UK is about 65%.

The treatment of invasive cervical cancer is stage-dependant. For early disease (stages Ib to IIa) radical surgery and radical radiotherapy are equally effective, leading to a cure for about 90% of women. For locally advanced disease (stages IIb to IVa) chemoradiation is generally the preferred treatment. The most successful drug in this context has been cisplatin, and a number of clinical trials have shown that combining it with radiation increases survival from about 60% to 80%, when compared with radiotherapy alone. To try and improve on these figures newer trials are looking at combining other cytotoxics with cisplatin, candidate drugs include paclitaxel and gemcitabine. The success of chemoradiation in bulky cervical cancer has led some clinicians to use it in earlier stage disease, either as an alternative or and adjunct to surgery.

For recurrent or advanced cervical cancer cisplatin has shown activity when used as a single agent, giving response rates of about 20%. When combined with paclitaxel this figure rises to about 35%, with median survival times of about 12 months. Other cytotoxic drugs that have shown activity in cervical cancer are gemcitabine, vinorelbine and topotecan but when combined with cisplatin none of these is superior to the combination of paclitaxel with cisplatin. Recently phase II studies have shown that bevacizumab has some activity in this disease and further trials are underway to clarify whether there is a role for this drug in cervical cancer.

Although they do not fall strictly under the heading of chemotherapy, it is important to mention that two vaccines are now available to protect against cervical cancer. More than 95% of cervical cancers are linked to human papilloma virus (HPV) infection, and about 70% are specifically linked to the type 16 and 18 HPV virus. Two vaccines, Gardasil and Cervarix have been developed against HPV 16 and 18 and their recent availability, and the introduction of mass vaccination programmes, offer the possibility of a dramatic reduction in cervical cancer incidence over the coming decades.

Suggestions for Further Reading

GSK Vaccine HPV-007 Study Group. Sustained efficacy and immuno-genicity of the human papillomavirus (HPV)-16/18AS04-adjuvaned vaccine: analysis of a randomised placebo-controlled trial up to 6.4 years. Lancet. 2009;374:1975–85.

Monk BJ, Sill MW, Burger RA, et al. Phase II trial of bevacizumab in the treatment of persistent or recurrent squamous cell carci-noma of the cervix. J Clin Oncol. 2009;27:1069–74.

Monk BJ, Sill MW, McMeekin DS ,et al. Phase III trial of four cispl-atin-containing doublet combinations in stage IVB, recurrent, or persistent cervical carcinoma: a Gynecologic Oncology Group study. J Clin Oncol. 2009;27:4649–55.

Munoz N, Manalastas R, Pitisuttithum P, et al. Safety, immunogenicity, and efficacy of quadrivalent human papillomavirus (types 6,11,16,18) recombinant vaccine in women aged 24–45 years: a randomised, double-blind trial. Lancet. 2009;373:1949–57.

Pectasides D, Kamposioras G, Papaxoinis G, Pectasides E. Chemotherapy for recurrent cervical cancer. Cancer Treat Rev. 2008;34:603–13.

Tewari KS, Monk BJ. Recent achievements and future developments in advanced and recurrent cervical cancer. Semin Oncol. 2009; 36:170–80.

Uterine Cancer

There are about 4,500 new cases of cancer of the womb each year in Britain, with 900 women dying annually of the disease. It is the fifth commonest cancer in women. The disease is rare before the age of 40 but rises rapidly in incidence between 40 and 50 remaining relatively constant thereafter until the age of 80, when its frequency declines. More than 85% of uterine cancers are adenocarcinomas arising from the endometrial lining of the organ. The remainder are either squamous cell carcinomas or uterine sarcomas. Between 70% and 80% of endometrial adenocarcinomas will be positive for progesterone receptors (PgR+), these are more likely to be present in well-differentiated tumours. The overall 5 year survival figure in the UK is about 76%.

The first line treatment for endometrial adenocarcinomas is surgery, which will usually involve a hysterectomy and bilateral salpingo-oophorectomy. More than 80% of these will be early, stage I or II lesions and there is no place for adjuvant therapy in these tumours. For stage III endometrial cancer radiotherapy has traditionally been the adjuvant therapy of choice but at least one clinical trial has suggested that chemotherapy, with the combination of cisplatin and doxorubicin may give better results and this has led to studies exploring the possibility of combining radiotherapy and chemotherapy to maximise the benefit. These trials are still in progress so the optimum adjuvant therapy for more advanced endometrial cancer remains to be established.

For women with metastatic or relapsed disease hormonal treatment with progestogens, such as medroxyprogesterone acetate or megestrol acetate, is often worthwhile and can lead to quite long-lasting remissions. For hormone resistant cancers cytotoxic therapy is an option. Studies have shown that the combination of cisplatin, doxorubicin and paclitaxel can produce responses in more than 50% of women and increase survival to around 15 months, compared to 8 or 9 months with single agent therapy. However, the triple drug regimen is quite toxic, and so using gentler single agent therapy with a platinum drug, taxane or anthracycline may still be preferable in some cases, especially as one is often dealing with an older population with significant comorbidities.

Suggestion for Further Reading

Carey MS, Gawlik, C, Fung-Kee M, et al. Systematic overview of systemic therapy for advanced or recurrent endometrial cancer. Gynecol Oncol. 2006;101:158–67.

Moxley KM, McMeekin. Endometrial cancer: a review of chemotherapy, drug resistance, and the search for new agents. Oncologist. 2010;15:1026–33.

Ray M, Fleming G. Management of advanced-stage and recurrent endometrial cancer. Semin Oncol. 2009;36:145–54.

Brain Tumours

Primary brain tumours make up about 1% of all cancers. They are a very diverse group of malignancies. Numerically the gliomas dominate (these are tumours arising from the supportive tissues within the brain, rather than neural tissue). Of the gliomas by far the most common are the astrocytomas, with nearly 4,000 new cases in adults each year in Britain, and about 3,000 deaths each year. Astrocytomas are also the commonest of all solid tumours in children. In adults the incidence of astrocytomas increases progressively with age, the average age at diagnosis being about 57. Astrocytomas are classified according to their histological appearance into either low grade (Grades I and II) or high grade (Grades III and IV) lesions. Grade III lesions are also known as anaplastic astrocytomas and grade IV astrocytomas are also known as glioblastoma multiforme. Low grade astrocytomas behave in a relatively benign fashion, and chemotherapy plays little or no part in their management, with surgery or radiotherapy being the definitive treatments. High grade astrocytomas, which account for more than 60% of these tumours, behave much more aggressively and carry a poor prognosis. Age is a strong predictor of outcome for high grade tumours, with about 50% of those under 40 surviving 18 months or more, whereas for people over 60 the figure is less than 10%. The overall 5 year survival is less than 5%.

With their aggressive behaviour and frequent rapid deterioration, many people with high grade astrocytomas, especially the elderly and those with a poor performance status, are not candidates for active treatment.

Many patients get dramatic short-term symptomatic relief from high-dose steroid therapy (dexamethasone, up to 16 mg daily), and for many people this, combined with general supportive care is the most appropriate treatment. For younger fitter patients surgery is often considered, but even when performed it is usually only possible to debulk the tumour rather than remove it completely. In this situation implantation of

Gliadel wafers at the time of operation may improve the outcome. These Gliadel implants are disc-shaped gel wafers, about 1 cm across. They contain the cytotoxic carmustine, and slowly dissolve in the brain, releasing the drug into the surrounding tissues over a period of 2–3 weeks.

For most people who have surgery this will be followed by radiotherapy to the brain, and radiotherapy is also the treatment option for those patients who were not suitable for surgery but are still fit enough for active treatment to be considered. Studies have suggested that adjuvant chemotherapy may be of value in selected patients, increasing survival by 2–3 months, and the two regimes that have been most widely used in the past are lomustine (CCNU), as a single agent, and PCV (procarbazine, lomustine and vincrtistine). These have now been widely superceded by temozolamide. When this drug is given during radiotherapy and for up to 6 months thereafter average survival times are increased by about 6 months, when compared to radiation alone. A completely different approach to adjuvant therapy that has been suggested is the use of chloroquine. This drug, usually used to treat malaria, augments the oxidative stress in glial cells caused by radiotherapy and thus enhances the effect of irradiation.

For people who relapse or have progressive disease, and have not had it before, temozolamide, is becoming the drug of choice, supplanting lomustine and PCV although these treatments remain options for those who have previously received temozolamide or who are no longer responding to it.

Suggestions for Further Reading

Munshi A. Chloroquine in glioblastoma – new horizons for an old drug. Cancer. 2009;115:2380–3.

Stupp R, Tonn J-C, Brada M, Pentheroudakis G. High grade malignant glioma: ESMO clinical practice guidelines for diagnosis, treatment and follow-up. Ann Oncol. 2010;21 Suppl 5:v190–3.

Wen PY, Kesari S. Malignant gliomas in adults. N Engl J Med. 2008;359:492–507.

Head and Neck Cancer

In Britain there are nearly 9,000 new cases of head and neck cancer each year, with some 2,700 deaths. Head and neck cancers comprise a very diverse group of tumours, but more than 80% are squamous cell carcinomas of the oral cavity, oropharynx or larynx. This discussion will be restricted to these lesions. They occur more often in men than women, at a ratio of 2.5:1. The average age at diagnosis is around 65. The overall 5 year survival rate for squamous cell cancers of the oral cavity and oropharynx is about 47%, whilst that for laryngeal cancers is about 65%.

Head and neck cancer is one area in oncology where the role of chemotherapy is developing particularly rapidly. This constantly evolving situation means that there are no universally agreed guidelines and practice is likely to vary quite significantly from centre to centre. As far as first line treatment is concerned either surgery or radiotherapy maybe appropriate depending on factors such as the site and size of the tumour and the general fitness of the patient.

In recent years clear evidence has emerged that the results of radiotherapy can be improved by giving concurrent chemotherapy (chemoradiation), particularly in people with locally advanced disease. Overall giving cytotoxic treatment alongside radiotherapy appears to increase the chance of cure by about 6%. This does, however, increase the risk of severe side-effects and so is generally avoided for those with very early stage disease (where less intensive treatment is still effective), or those who are less fit or who have metastatic disease. Cisplatin is the most widely used cytotoxic in combination with radiation. However, trial data has also shown that combining the EGFR antagonist cetuximab with radiotherapy also increases survival, compared to radiotherapy alone, without a significant increase in toxicity. As yet there are no data comparing chemoradiation with cisplatin with chemoradiation with cetuximab, but the latter does appear to offer a less toxic regimen for less fit patients. These results also offer the possibility of exploring the effect of combining cetuximab with cisplatin-based chemoradiation.

Giving conventional adjuvant cytotoxic chemotherapy after surgery or radiotherapy has not been shown to clearly improve long-term survival. However, the observation that when patients relapse after chemoradiation it is usually because of distant metastases, rather than local recurrence of the disease, has led to the suggestion that induction, or neo-adjuvant, chemotherapy, given prior to the chemoradiation might improve the long-term results. Clinical trials using combinations of either paclitaxel or docetaxel with cisplatin and fluorouracil as induction therapies have shown promising results. For patients with locally advanced, bulky disease, neo-adjuvant therapy may also act as a good predictor of response to radiotherapy, with patients achieving a good partial response being likely to benefit from intensive chemoradiation whereas those who show no obvious tumour shrinkage are unlikely to benefit from this intensive regimen and should probably be offered the gentler option of radiotherapy alone.

For people who do relapse with local recurrence then salvage surgical measures with either conventional resections or laser surgery may be helpful. As far as chemotherapy is concerned cytotoxic treatment is of limited value but the combination of cisplatin and fluorouracil is often used. For those patients who achieve a good response, and go on to relapse more than 3 months after completion of their treatment, then second line therapy with cytotoxics such as methotrexate or one of the taxanes may be worth a try.

Suggestions for Further Reading

Argiris A, Karamouzis MV, Raben D, Ferris RL. Head and neck cancer. Lancet. 2008;371:1695–709.

Gold KA, Lee H-Y. Kim ES. Targeted therapies in squamous cell carcinoma of the head and neck. Cancer. 2009;115:922–35.

Mehanna H, West CML, Nutting C, Paleri P. Head and neck cancer. Part 1: epidemiology, presentation and prevention. Br Med J. 2010; 341:c4684.

Mehanna H, West CML, Nutting C, Paleri P. Head and neck cancer. Part 2: treatment and prognostic factors. Ibid c4690.

Skin Cancer

The principal types of skin cancer are basal cell carcinomas, squamous cell carcinomas and malignant melanoma. The great majority of skin cancers in the UK are either basal or squamous cell carcinomas, with more than 100,000 cases being diagnosed each year. Chemotherapy plays virtually no part in the management of these cancers, but occasionally topical application of fluorouracil cream (in concentrations of 0.5–5%) may be recommended for very superficial basal cell carcinomas.

Each year in Britain there are almost 12,000 new cases of malignant melanoma, making it the eighth commonest cancer in the UK. There are 1,800 deaths annually from malignant melanoma in Britain. The first line management of localised melanoma is surgery, with a wide local excision. The 5 year survival rate for men is about 80% and for women it is about 90%.

Numerous clinical trials have explored the role of adjuvant chemotherapy for the more advanced stages of localised disease, but none has yet shown a convincing benefit. For patients who are keen to explore adjuvant therapy the recommendation should be for them to enter an appropriate clinical trial.

Metastatic melanoma is a relatively chemoresistant disease. The drug which has been most extensively explored in this indication is the cytotoxic dacarbazine (DTIC). Used as a single agent this has produced partial response rates ranging from 15% to 30%, with complete responses in 3–5% of patients. However, there is no convincing evidence that treatment leads to any increase in survival. Similarly although some trials combining DTIC with other cytotoxics, or interferon, have claimed higher response rates there are still no clear data to support the view that life-expectancy is prolonged, compared to giving best supportive care.

This gloomy situation has improved recently with the introduction of two drugs which, for the first time, have actually shown an increase in survival in metastatic melanoma. The drugs are ipilimumab and vemurafenib. Ipilimumab is a monoclonal antibody, given by intravenous infusion, which stimulates the immune system by blocking cytotoxic T-lymphocyte-associated antigen four and appears to increase median survival by about 4 months. Vemurafenib is an oral agent which targets a specific gene mutation (the BRAF V600E mutation) which is carried by about 50% of melanoma patients. In those who have the mutation about 50% have a response to vemurafenib and life expectancy does appear to be prolonged but by how much is uncertain at the present time.

Suggestions for Further Reading

Chapman PB, Hauschild A, Robert C, et al. Improved survival with vemurafenib in melanoma with BRAF V600E mutation. N Engl J Med. 2011;364:2507–16.

Hodi FS, O'Day SJ, McDermott DF, et al. Improved survival with ipilimumab in patients with metastatic melanoma. N Engl J Med. 2010;363:711–23.

NICE. Improving Outcomes for People with Skin Cancers Including Melanoma. Department of Health. 2006.

Soft Tissue Sarcomas

There are about 2,200 new cases of soft tissue sarcoma each year in Britain, making up about 1% of all cancers. Just under 1,000 people die annually of the disease. The average age at the time of diagnosis is the early 60s, although these tumours may occur at any age. Soft tissue sarcomas make up a very diverse group of cancers (Table 3.3). Fifty percent of these growths occur in the limbs, 40% in the trunk or retroperitoneum, and 10% in the head and neck. The overall 5 year survival figure in the UK is between 50% and 60%, although the figures do vary considerably for different tumour types and sites, for example retroperitoneal soft tissue sarcomas tend to have a poorer outlook, largely because of their later presentation. The size and histological grade of the sarcoma are also important prognostic features with larger tumours,

TABLE 3.3 Relative incidence of soft tissue sarcoma[a]

	All sites (%)	Soft tissues only (%)
Leiomyosarcoma	24	12
Malignant fibrous histiocytoma	17	25
Liposarcoma	12	24
Dermatofibrosarcoma	11	2
Rhabdomysarcoma	5	5
Angiosarcoma	4	4
Nerve sheath tumours	4	6
Fibrosarcoma	4	5

[a]Soft tissue sarcomas may occur either in specific organs or in the soft tissues, and the incidence of the different types of sarcoma differs between the two sites. Approximately 50% of the sarcomas occur in soft tissues and 50% in specific organs. Among the latter the commonest are skin (28%), uterus (14%), the retroperitoneum (14%), stomach (8%), and small intestine (6%)

>5 cm, and high grade, grade III, cancers (which account for about 50% of these growths), faring worse.

Whenever possible surgery is the treatment of choice for these lesions, with removal of the primary cancer and a margin of at least 2 cm of surrounding normal tissue. When there is doubt about the completeness of the excision, or for larger, high grade lesions then post-operative radiotherapy is usually recommended.

Results suggest that adjuvant chemotherapy is of limited value. Local and distant relapse may be delayed by treatment but there are no convincing data that overall survival is increased. Clinical trials in this area are still continuing, particularly for larger lesions. Neoadjuvant, pre-operative chemotherapy is sometimes used for larger sarcomas, to try and improve the surgical outcome.

Soft tissue sarcomas tend to spread predominantly to the lungs, and resection of isolated lung metastatases may sometimes be a treatment option in advanced disease. Cytotoxic chemotherapy is of only limited value. The most active agents are doxorubicin and ifosfamide. When used as single agents they have a response rate of about 20%. Given in combination with dacarbazine, this figure rises to between 30% and 35%, but this is quite an aggressive regimen, most suitable for younger fitter patients. For those people who respond their life expectancy may be increased by a few months. Recently the alkylating agent trabectedin has been approved for use in people who relapse after ifosfamide or doxorubicin therapy and this drug may add a further few months to survival times.

One type of soft tissue sarcoma that merits special mention is gastrointestinal stromal tumour (GIST). These have been distinguished as a separate entity in the last decade, many previously being considered leiomyosarcomas. These are the commonest sarcoma of the gastrointestinal tract, with about 800 new cases in Britain each year. Surgery is the primary treatment wherever possible. Conventional cytotoxics are ineffective for more advanced stages of the disease, but more than 80% of these cancers carry a KIT gene mutation and are susceptible to the tyrosine kinase inhibitor imatinib. As a result these patients with advanced disease will gain a response lasting in excess of 2 years on average, and their median 5 year survival will be about 5 years, compared with only 1 year before imatinib was introduced. Studies have also been done looking at the use of imatinib in the adjuvant setting, following surgery. There is some evidence that it may reduce the risk of relapse but at the present time in the UK it has not been approved in this indication by NICE. Another tyrosine kinase inhibitor, sunitinib, is currently being evaluated for use in patients with relapsed or resistant GIST following imatinib therapy.

Suggestions for Further Reading

Clark MA, Fisher C, Judson I, Thomas JM. Soft-tissue sarcomas in adults. N Engl J Med. 2005;353:701–11.

DeMatteo RP, Ballman KV, Antonescu CR, et al. Adjuvant imatinib mesylate after resection of localized primary gastro-intestinal stromal tumour: a randomized, double-blind trial. Lancet. 2009; 373:1097–104.

NICE technology appraisal guidance 196. Imatinib for the adjuvant treatment of gastrointestinal stromal tumours. NICE. 2010.

Toro JR, Travis LB, Wu HJ, et al. Incidence patterns of soft tissue sarcoma, regardless of primary site, in the surveillance, epidemiology and end results program, 1978–2001: an analysis of 26,758 cases. Int J Cancer. 2006;119:2922–30.

Trabectedin for the treatment of advanced soft tissue sarcomas. NICE technology appraisal guidance 185. NICE. 2010.

Primary Bone Sarcomas

There are about 450 new cases of bone sarcomas each year in Britain, making up about 0.2% of all cancers. About 200 people die annually of the disease. The majority of these cancers occur between the ages of 10 and 20, although there is a second peak in the over 60s which accounts for about 10% of cases. Primary bone tumours are commoner in men than women with a ratio of 3:2. The overall 5 year survival figure in the UK is just over 50%. Osteosarcomas are the commonest type of primary bone sarcoma, other types are Ewing's sarcoma, chondrosarcoma and spindle cell sarcomas (the latter being made up of a variety of tumour types, generally behaving in a similar way to osteosarcoma, and occurring in older people).

For osteosarcomas treatment is based on a combination of surgery and chemotherapy. Surgery is aimed at removing the primary tumour, which may involve an amputation. Cytotoxic chemotherapy is given pre-operatively (neoadjuvant therapy), to shrink the primary lesion, facilitating surgery, and is continued as post-operative adjuvant therapy. The most widely used treatment schedule is based on giving cisplatin, doxorubicin and high dose methotrexate followed by leucovorin rescue, ifosfamide is sometimes added to this regimen. A recent development has been the addition of the immunomodulator mifamurtide to the treatment protocol for young people, under the age of 30, and this appears to increase the chance of cure by about 10%.

For Ewing's sarcoma radiotherapy or surgery are used to treat the primary growth but adjuvant cytotoxic chemotherapy is then essential to maximise the chance of cure. In the UK and Europe favoured treatment schedules are vincristine, ifosfamide, doxorubicin and etoposide (VIDE) given every 3 weeks for six courses, or vincristine, ifosfamide and dactinomycin (VIA) given every 3 weeks for eight courses. In the North America combinations of either vincristine, doxorubicin and cyclophosphamide, or ifosfamide and etoposide tend to be preferred.

Treatment of chondrosarcomas and spindle cell sarcomas tends to be similar to that of osteosarcoma, although the chemotherapy schedules may be less intense as it is generally an older group of patients who are being treated.

Suggestions for Further Reading

Balamuth NJ, Womer RB. Ewing's sarcoma. Lancet Oncol. 2010; 11:184–92.

Geller DS, Gorlick R. Osteosarcoma: a review of diagnosis, management and treatment strategies. Clin Adv Hematol Oncol. 2010;8:705–18.

NICE technology appraisal guidance 235. Mifamurtide for the treatment of osteosarcoma. NICE. 2011.

Haematological Cancer

Acute Lymphoblastic Leukaemia

Acute lymphoblastic leukaemia (ALL) is a disease of progenitor cells for either B-cell or T-cell lymphocytes. In ALL these cells escape from normal growth control mechanisms and lose the ability to differentiate remaining as primitive blast cells, appearing in the peripheral blood and infiltrating the bone marrow.

There are about 550 new cases of ALL each year in Britain. Of these about two thirds are in children and adolescents, with a peak age of 3–4 years. In adults the median age

at diagnosis ranges from 25 to 37, this reflects a high incidence in young adults, and a second peak occurring in those
over 75.

Progressive improvements in chemotherapy and supportive care over the last 50 years mean that in children the overall cure rate is in excess of 80%. Unfortunately the figure is
far worse in adults, being about 40%. Age is a strong prognostic factor in adults, with older people faring worse. About
25% of adults, and 5% of children, with ALL will have
leukaemic cells which carry the Philadelphia chromosome
(see page 155).

There are a number of different subtypes of ALL and
there are subtle differences in the treatment for each of these
but in general for both adults and children there are four
components to management: remission induction, consolidation or intensification, maintenance and CNS prophylaxis.

For children remission induction typically involves the use
of a steroid (either prednisone, prednisolone, or dexamethasone), vincristine and asparaginase. For those with a poor
prognosis, and most young adults, an anthracycline, usually
daunorubicin will be added. For those adults with the
Philadelphia chromosome the tyrosine kinase inhibitor, imatinib is added to their drug regimen. Treatment extends over
4–6 weeks, with the aim of destroying 99% or more of the leukaemic cells. The treatment is intensive and requires rigorous
supportive care with red cell and platelet transfusions and
infection prophylaxis, so it is done on an in-patient basis. The
response to remission induction is a strong prognostic marker,
with those who fail to gain a complete remission within 4
weeks having a poor outlook, however more than 95% of children and 80–90% of adults will go into remission.

For those who achieve a remission the next stage is
intensification, or consolidation. This involves a variety of different regimens depending on the patient's age and the precise subtype of ALL. Typical treatments include high-dose
methotrexate with mercaptopurine, or high-dose asparaginase with vincristine and a steroid, or a repeat of the original
induction regimen. This phase usually lasts from 4 to 8 weeks.

An alternative at this stage, particularly for young adults, is an allogeneic stem-cell transplant.

Maintenance, or continuation therapy involves gentler, long-term chemotherapy, for between 2 and 3 years. The most widely used combination is daily oral mercaptopurine with weekly oral methotrexate. Adults with the Philadelphia chromosome will also continue imatinib.

Unless treatment is given between 30% and 50% of people who achieve a remission will relapse with CNS involvement by their leukaemia. It is impossible to predict who will develop this problem so treatment known as 'CNS prophylaxis' is almost universally given. This used to involve radiotherapy to the brain and spinal cord, but carried the risk of long-term complications including a degree of mental impairment and pituitary damage, so is now generally avoided. The usual alternative is intrathecal administration of methotrexate (see page 51). Depending on individual treatment protocols this may be given as part of remission induction, or intensification, or maintenance, or at all three stages of treatment.

Suggestion for Further Reading

Pui C-H, Evans WE. Treatment of acute lymphoblastic leukemia. N Engl J Med. 2006;354:166–78.

Pui C-H, Robison LL. Acute lymphoblastic leukaemia. Lancet. 2008;371:1030–43.

Acute Myeloid Leukaemia

Acute myeloid leukaemia (AML) is a disease of bone marrow stem cells, which produce red blood cells, neutrophils and platelets. In AML these cells escape from normal growth control mechanisms and lose the ability to differentiate remaining as primitive blast cells. When the bone marrow contains more than 20% of blast cells then AML is diagnosed. Failure of red cell and platelet formation lead to anaemia and bleeding disorders and the absence of mature neutrophils leads to infection, which is the usual cause of death.

There are about 2,000 new cases of AML each year in Britain, with an average at diagnosis of 70. There are a number of different types of AML and 55% of people with the disease show specific cytogenetic abnormalities in their blast cells which allow not only for precise classification of their AML subtype but also give a guide to prognosis. Age is a major prognostic factor, with people over 55–60 faring far worse than younger adults. Performance status, and a number of biochemical measures, such as serum albumin, bilirubin and creatinine levels also influence outcome.

For younger adults, below the age of 60, the cornerstone of treatment is induction of complete remission which typically relies on a regimen of the cytotoxics daunorubicin (given intravenously on three consecutive days) and cytarabine (given by continuous intravenous infusion for 7–10 days). This combination will produce a complete remission (defined as <5% blasts in the bone marrow) in 65–75% of people. Other drugs which may be used in remission induction are etoposide, fludarabine and idarubicin. In one specific type of AML – acute promyelocytic leukaemia – the drug all-trans retinoic acid, vitamin A, is highly effective and is combined with an anthracycline cytotoxic in remission induction.

Once a remission has been achieved the next stage is consolidation therapy, which for good and intermediate prognosis individuals involves one of a number of regimens. Among the commonest of these are high dose cytarabine therapy or a repeat of two courses of induction therapy, followed by a course of m-amsacrine, cytarabine and etoposide followed by a final course of mitoxantrone and cytarabine. Once again all-trans retinoic acid is of value in acute promyelocytic leukaemia. Unlike acute lymphoblastic leukaemia there is no benefit in giving long-term maintenance therapy. For the poor risk group options include allogeneic stem cell transplants or experimental therapies. Depending on prognostic factors the overall cure rate for this age group lies between 20% and 75%.

The place of targeted therapies in AML is unclear. Clinical trials have focused on adding gemtuzumab to conventional chemotherapy. Gemtuzumab is a conjugate of a monoclonal antibody, which targets the CD33 protein on the leukaemic cells, and a cytotoxic called calicheamicin. A major study in the USA showed that the drug not only failed to increase the remission rate but caused a number of life-threatening toxicities. However, two very recent European trials, using a different dosing schedule for the drug have actually shown an increase in survival figures with acceptable toxicity.

For older patients options include standard daunorubicin-cytarabine, possibly with gemtuzumab, experimental therapy or supportive care. Overall, however, the outcomes are disappointing with less than 10% of people being cured, and the average survival only stretching to 10 months. Certainly in the USA figures suggest of those people over 65 with AML only one third get chemotherapy and the overall median survival in this age group is only 3 months.

Suggestions for Further Reading

British Committee for Standards in Haematology. Guidelines on the management of acute myeloid leukaemia in adults. Br J Haematol. 2006;135:450–74.

Dohner H, Estey EH, Amodori S, et al. Diagnosis and management of acute myeloid leukemia in adults: recommendations from an international panel on behalf of European LeukemiaNet. Blood. 2010;115:453–74.

Estey E, Dohner H. Acute myeloid leukaemia. Lancet. 2006;368: 1894–907.

Chronic Myeloid Leukaemia

As with acute myeloid leukaemia the underlying abnormality is overproduction of bone marrow stem cells. Ninety-five percent of people with chronic myeloid leukemia (CML) have a translocation between chromosomes 9 and 22, producing what is known as the Philadelphia chromosome. This translocation produces a fusion gene, BCR-ABL, which in turn generates a specific tyrosine kinase pathway which stimulates cell division.

There are about 650 new cases of CML in Britain each year, with an average of onset of 66 (although about 2% of cases occur in children). The disease goes through three phases. Firstly there is the chronic phase, which lasts about 3–5 years. Often a raised white cell count is the only abnormality during this time and symptoms are few, the condition frequently being diagnosed as the result of a routine blood test. This is followed by the accelerated phase which lasts anywhere from 2 to 15 months. During this time anaemia and splenomegaly develop causing symptoms of tiredness and abdominal discomfort, and an increased risk of infection and bleeding problems. Finally there is the blast crisis which lasts just a few months. This is essentially a transformation to an acute myeloid leukaemia, and is invariably fatal.

An allogeneic stem cell transplant is the only curative option for CML but most patients are too old for this to be considered. Over the last decade the drug treatment of CML has been transformed by the discovery of imatinib (Glivec). This is a signal transduction inhibitor which specifically blocks BCR-ABL tyrosine kinase activity. When given to people in the chronic phase of CML at a dose of 200 mg bd, more than 95% gain a response with nearly 90% still being alive after 5 years. Treatment with imatinib is continued indefinitely as even complete responders appear to be at risk of relapse if the drug is stopped. In order to be effective imatinib must be given as soon as possible after a diagnosis is made, treatment should be initiated in the chronic phase of the disease, even though there may be no symptoms, and not delayed until the condition progresses.

Recent randomised clinical trials with two of the newer BCR-ABL tyrosine kinase inhibitors, dasatinib and nilotinib, indicate that they are even more effective than imatinib in inducing remissions, including complete molecular remissions, with disappearance of all traces of the BCR-ABL gene from the blood. Whether these benefits are retained in the long-term remains to be seen and this uncertainty, together with economic concerns over the cost of the newer agents means that in most situations imatinib remains the first choice therapy, but nilotinib and dasatinib do offer options for people who cannot tolerate imatinib or become resistant to it.

Treatment options for people who relapse on imatinib include interferon, cytotoxic chemotherapy with drugs like hydroxyurea (also known as hydroxycarbamide), busulphan, or cytarabine, or an allogeneic stem cell transplant, but the outcomes are uncertain.

Suggestions for Further Reading

Hehlmann R, Hochaus A, Baccarani M. Chronic myeloid leukaemia. Lancet. 2007;370:342–50.

Kantarjian H, Shah NP, Hochaus A, et al. Dasatinib versus imatinib in newly diagnosed chronic-phase chronic myeloid leukemia. N Engl J Med. 2010;362:2260–9.

Saglio G, Kim D-W, Issaragrisil S, et al. Nilotinib versus imatinib for newly diagnosed chronic myeloid leukemia. N Engl J Med. 2010; 362:2251–9.

Chronic Lymphocytic Leukaemia

In chronic lymphocytic leukaemia (CLL) the underlying abnormality is an overproduction of lymphocytes, which appear in the bone marrow, the circulating blood and as lymph node masses. Rather confusingly CLL is also be classified as form of low grade non-Hodgkin lymphoma.

There are about 4,500 new cases of CLL each year in Britain. The average age of onset is between 65 and 70. The overall median life-expectancy from the time of diagnosis is around 10 years, but there are wide individual variations. Between 75% and 80% of cases are asymptomatic and discovered as the result of routine blood tests, in the remainder the presenting symptoms are usually either enlarged lymph nodes, or tiredness due to anaemia.

The disease is normally indolent and asymptomatic patients often require no treatment initially. Indications for starting therapy include progressive bone marrow failure (with either anaemia or thrombocytopenia), enlarging lymph nodes or progressive splenomegaly, a rapid increase in the number of circulating lymphocytes, or the onset of systemic symptoms such as weight loss or fever.

In contrast to CML there is no good evidence that treatment during the indolent phase of the disease improves the outcome so a watch and wait policy is usually appropriate, keeping treatment in reserve until symptoms develop. Traditionally first line active treatment has been based on single agent cytotoxic chemotherapy with the main choices being either chlorambucil, or fludarabine. Both these agents can be given orally, and result in remissions in 75–80% of patients, with about 30–40% of the being complete remissions, median survivals at 5 years are about 50%. On relapse further responses can often be obtained by either rechallenging with the original drug, or changing from one to the other. Other drugs that may be used are bendamustine and cladribine. This approach is still applicable for elderly, less fit people but for younger fitter patients other treatments are evolving.

In selected cases an allogeneic transplant is an option, and offers the only chance of cure, although the procedure is not without its risks and carries a mortality of about 20%. For most younger fitter people the preferred treatment will be combination therapy with cytotoxic drugs and a monoclonal antibody, the most widely used combinations being fludarabine, cyclophosphamide and rituximab (FCR) or bendamustine and rituximab.

A special subgroup of patients can be defined as being 'high risk' and they have a deletion on chromosome 17 which renders them less sensitive to conventional treatments. If they are not suitable for an allogeneic transplant then monotherapy with the monoclonal antibody alemtuzumab or the FCR regimen can be tried but most people will go into clinical trials attempting to define the optimum therapy in this situation.

The enlarged lymph node masses which occur in CLL are very sensitive to radiotherapy and this may also be used to help control the disease in its more advanced stages. High dose steroid therapy may also be useful at this time.

Suggestion for Further Reading

Garcia-Escobar I, Sepulveda J, Castellano D, Cortes-Funes H. Therapeutic management of chronic lymphocytic leukemia. State of the art and future perspectives. Crit Rev Oncol Hematol. 2011;80:100–13.

Hallek M, Pflug N. State of the art treatment for chronic lymphocytic leukemia. Blood Rev. 2011;25:1–9.

Lymphomas

Lymphomas are traditionally divided into Hodgkin lymphoma, and non-Hodgkin lymphomas (NHL). Hodgkin lymphoma is named after the English pathologist, Thomas Hodgkin who first described the disease in the 1832, and is distinguished from other lymphomas by the presence of a specific type of abnormal B-lymphocyte: the Reed-Sternberg cell.

Hodgkin Lymphoma

There are about 1,400 new cases of Hodgkin lymphoma each year In Britain. The peak age of incidence is in young adults, although people of any age may be affected. Discovery of a swollen lymph node mass is the usual presenting feature but occasionally systemic symptoms: weight loss, fever, generalised itching, may dominate the picture. Forty years ago the condition was almost universally fatal but as the result firstly of wide-field radiotherapy, and then of developments in combination chemotherapy the overall cure rate is now in excess of 75%.

The choice of treatment depends on the specific cellular sub-type of Hodgkin lymphoma (Table 3.4), the stage of the disease (Table 3.5), and other prognostic factors. From these four subgroups can be identified:

Early favourable disease: non-bulky stage IA or II A. These patients used to be treated by wide field radiotherapy but increasing concerns about the risk of second malignancies and other long-term complications has led to an increasing preference for cytotoxic chemotherapy. Drug regimens that have

TABLE 3.4 Hodgkin lymphoma: cellular classification

Classical Hodgkin lymphoma

Nodular sclerosis

Mixed-cellularity

Lymphocyte depleted

Lymphocyte-rich classical

Nodular lymphocyte-predominant HL

This is a more indolent form of the disease, with a tendency to recur.

TABLE 3.5 The staging of Hodgkin lymphoma (simplified)

I. Involvement of a single lymph node region

II. Involvement of two or more lymph node regions on the same side of the diaphragm

III. Involvement of lymph node regions on both sides of the diaphragm

IV. Multifocal involvement of one or more extralymphatic organs

These stages may be subclassified with the suffix A or B. The B designation is given to people with one or more of the following symptoms:

unexplained weight loss of more than 10%

unexplained fever with temperatures above 38°C

drenching night sweats

been used include MOPP (nitrogen mustard, vincristine, procarbazine and prednisone), BEACOPP (bleomycin, etoposide, doxorubicin, cyclophosphamide, vincristine, procarbazine and prednisone), and ABVD (doxorubicin, bleomycin, vinblastine and dacarbazine). Although MOPP was the pioneer combination which revolutionised the outcome in Hodgkin lymphoma both it and BEACOPP almost always lead to infertility, and also carry about a 3% risk of developing secondary acute leukaemia. By contrast ABVD has little effect on fertility and has <1% risk of leukaemia, so has become the preferred treatment. For these patients the treatment options are either 4–6 courses of ABVD, or four courses of ABVD followed by radiotherapy to the involved lymph node sites, although recent trial results have queried the need for radiation.

Early unfavourable disease: stage IA or IIA with B symptoms, bulky disease or other adverse prognostic factors. Bulky disease is defined as lymph node masses greater than 10 cm in diameter, or mediastinal disease greater than one 33% of the thoracic diameter. The usually choice of treatment here is either 4–6 cycles of ABVD, or four cycles of ABVD followed by radiotherapy to the involved lymph node sites. These will result in a cure rate in excess of 80%.

Advanced favourable disease: stage III or IV disease with few adverse prognostic factors. The most widely used regimen is 6–8 cycles of ABVD, which may be followed by local radiotherapy if there was bulky disease. This will result in a cure rate of about 60%.

Advanced unfavourable disease: stage III or IV with poor prognostic factors. Options here include either 6–8 cycles of ABVD, or 6–8 cycles of BEACOPP. These will give a cure rate of up to 50%.

Non-Hodgkin Lymphoma

These are a diverse group of cancers and over the last 30 years more than 25 different systems have been suggested for their classification. Currently the most widely accepted system is the REAL/WHO classification. From a clinical viewpoint these various conditions can be grouped into indolent, or low grade NHL, or aggressive, or high grade NHL (Table 3.6). Between 60% and 80% of people with low grade NHL will survive 10 years or more and about 60% of those with high grade disease will be cured.

There are about 8,000 new cases of low grade NHL, and nearly 4,000 of high grade NHL, each year in Britain, and the incidence of the disease is steadily increasing at a rate of about 3% per year. Overall NHL is the sixth commonest cancer in the UK. Although the average age of onset is 55–60 people of any age may be affected. The clinical presentations vary widely but the discovery of enlarged lymph node masses

TABLE 3.6 Principal types of non-Hodgkin lymphoma, and their incidence

Low grade	
B-cell cancers	
Follicular lymphoma	22%
Extranodal marginal zone lymphoma (MALT lymphoma)	8%
B-cell small lymphocytic lymphoma/chronic lymphocytic leukaemia	7%
Nodal marginal zone lymphoma	2%
Lymphoplasmacytic lymphoma/ Waldentrom's macroglobulinaemia	1%
High grade	
B-cell cancers	
Diffuse large B-cell lymphoma	33%
Mantle cell lymphoma	6%
Burkitt's lymphoma	2%
T-cell cancers	
Mature (peripheral) T-cell neoplasms	8%
Precursor T-lymphoblastic lymphoma/ leukaemia	2%
Primary systemic anaplastic large cell lymphoma	2%

is the most common. The staging system for NHL is similar to that for Hodgkin lymphoma, although most people present with stage III or IV disease.

Although treatment varies with the individual type of NHL the broad principles of managing low grade and high grade disease are as follows:

Low grade disease: in a few instances the disease will be truly localised, confined to one or two groups of lymph nodes, and in this situation radiotherapy may result in a cure. In all other situations low grade NHL is usually incurable, although the disease often progresses very slowly, with an overall median survival of about 10 years. Because of its slow progression and relative lack of symptoms some people may need no immediate treatment, and can enter a policy of watchful waiting, being regularly monitored with treatment being reserved until there are clear signs of disease progression. When treatment is needed cytotoxic chemotherapy is the usual choice, and options include oral chlorambucil as a single agent, or combination regimens with either CVP (cyclophosphamide, vincristine and prednisone), or CHOP (cyclophosphamide, doxorubicin, vincristine, and prednisone). There is now good evidence that adding the monoclonal antibody rituximab to any of these regimens increases the chance of remission and for those people who gain a benefit maintenance therapy with rituximab for up to 2 years has been shown to delay relapse and improve overall survival. Rituximab binds to a protein called CD20 which is found on the surface of normal and malignant B-cell lymphocytes. Malignant B-cell lymphocytes are the dominant cancer cell type in most types of low grade NHL. Although these drugs will bring about complete remissions for many people the disease will ultimately recur and re-treatment will be necessary.

High grade NHL: paradoxically, although it is more aggressive, the chances of a cure are greater with high grade than low grade NHL, with between 30% and 60% of people surviving long-term. Chemotherapy is the cornerstone of treatment with either CHOP, or R-CHOP (CHOP+ rituximab) for 4–8 courses. For some patients this may be followed by radiotherapy to the involved lymph node areas. For some younger patients, who have gone into remission but who are considered to be at high risk of relapse, bone marrow or stem cell transplantation may be considered.

Suggestions for Further Reading

Armitage JO. Early-stage Hodgkin's lymphoma. N Engl J Med. 2010;363:653–62.

Canellos GP, Niedzwiecki D, Johnson JL. Long-term follow-up of survival in Hodgkin's lymphoma. N Engl J Med. 2009;361:2390–1.

Lim SH, Johnson WM. Chemotherapy: advanced Hodgkin lymphoma – balancing toxicity and cure. Nat Rev Clin Oncol. 2011;8:634–6.

Lowry L, Hoskin P, Linch D. Developments in the management of Hodgkin's lymphoma. Lancet. 2010;375:786–8.

Meyer RM, Gospodarowicz MK, Connors JM, et al. ABVD alone versus radiation-based therapy in limited stage Hodgkin's lymphoma. N Engl J Med. 2012;366:399–408.

McNamara C. Evolution of first-line therapy for symptomatic advanced-stage follicular lymphoma. Oncol News. 2012;6:200–1.

NICE Technology Appraisal Guidance 137. Rituximab for the treatment of relapsed or refractory stage III or IV follicular non-Hodgkin's lymphoma. NICE. 2008.

Multiple Myeloma

The underlying abnormality in multiple myeloma is a proliferation of abnormal plasma cells (plasma cells are derived from B-lymphocytes, and are responsible for antibody production). These settle in the bone marrow and cause destruction of the surrounding bone, leading to pain and fractures. Normal plasma cells are involved in antibody formation and produce immunoglobulins, their malignant counterparts usually produce abnormal amounts of specific immunoglobulins and the high concentrations of these can lead to complications such as renal failure.

There are about 3,300 new cases of multiple myeloma each year in Britain. The median age at presentation is about 70, and fewer than 2% of patients are diagnosed under 40. Bone pain is the commonest presenting symptom. The condition is incurable but survival times are very variable, ranging from a few months to more than 20 years.

Some people may be asymptomatic when multiple myeloma is first diagnosed, and for them it is often safe to withhold treatment until there is evidence of disease progression, which may be anywhere from 1 to 3 years. Once treatment is indicated the choice of therapy is determined by a number of factors, including the patient's age and general fitness.

For younger patients, below the ages of 55–65, some form of high-dose chemotherapy and a stem cell transplant may be considered. In this situation the induction treatment has relied on cytotoxic drug combinations such as VAD (vincristine, doxorubicin and dexamethasone), but there is evidence from a number of trials that adding one of the newer agents such as thalidomide, lenalidomide or bortezomib to this regimen can improve the outcome increasing the chance of 5 year survival to over 50%. As yet no single regimen has emerged as the treatment of choice.

The majority of people, however, a stem cell transplant is not going to be an option because of their age and fitness. In this situation the traditional approach is gentler oral treatment with melphalan and prednisolone. Once again recent trials have shown that adding either thalidomide, lenalidomide or bortezomib to this combination boosts complete response rates and 3 year survival to over 80%.

Bone pain is a major problem in multiple myeloma. Successful chemotherapy often eases the problem but for those people where symptoms persist localised radiotherapy (usually only requiring a single low dose treatment) or bisphosphonates given orally or by intravenous infusions every 4–6 weeks may be very beneficial. Bisphosphonates also help reduce the risk of bone fractures and spinal cord compression.

Suggestions for Further Reading

Gay F, Palumbo A. Management of older patients with myeloma. Blood Rev. 2011;25:65–73.

Hicks LK, Haynes AE, Reece DE. A meta-analysis and systematic review of thalidomide for patients with previously untreated multiple myeloma. Cancer Treat Rev. 2008;34:442–52.

Raab MS, Podar K, Breitkreutz I, et al. Multiple myeloma. Lancet. 2009;374:324–39.

San Miguel JF, Schlag R, Khuageva NK, et al. Bortezomib plus melphalan and prednisone for initial treatment of multiple myeloma. N Engl J Med. 2008;359:906–17.

Appendix

Appendix A: Chemotherapeutic Agents and Their Trade Names

Alkylating agents

Bendamustine (Levact)

Busulfan (Myleran, Busilvex)

Carmustine, BCNU (BiCNU, Gliadel wafers)

Chlorambucil (Leukeran)

Cyclophosphamide (Endoxana)

Dacarbazine, DTIC

Ifosfamide (Mitoxana)

Melphalan (Alkeran)

Mitomycin (Mitomycin C Kyowa)

Temozolamide (Temodal)

Trabectidin (Yondelis)

Platinum analogues

Carboplatin (Paraplatin)

Oxaliplatin (Eloxatin)

Antimetabolites

Capecitabine (Xeloda)

Cladribine (Leustat, Litak)

Cytarabine (lipid formulation: DepoCyte)

Fludarabine (Fludara)

Mercaptopurine (Puri-nethol)

Pemetrexed (Alimta)

Pentostatin (Nipent)

Raltitrexed (Tomudex)

T. Priestman, *Cancer Chemotherapy in Clinical Practice,*
DOI 10.1007/978-0-85729-727-3,
© Springer-Verlag London 2012

Fluorouracil (topical: Efudix)

Tegafur with uracil
(Uftoral)

Gemcitabine (Gemzar)

Thioguanine, tioguanine
(Lanvis)

Hydroxyurea (Hydrea)

Topoisomerase I inhibitors

Irinotecan (Campto)

Topotecan (Hycamtin)

Topoisomerase II inhibitors

Amsacrine (Amisidine)

Etoposide (Etophos,
Vepesid)

Daunorubicin (lipid formulation:
DaunoXome)

Idarubicin (Zavedos)

Doxorubicin (Adriamycin, lipid
formulation: Caelyx, Myocet)

Mitoxantrone (Onkotrone,
Mitoxantrone)

Epirubicin (Pharmorubicin)

Cytotoxic antibiotics

Bleomycin (Bleomycin)

Dactinomycin,
actinomycin D (Cosmogen
Lyovac)

Anti-microtubule drugs

Cabazitaxel (Jevtana)

Vincristine (Oncovin)

Docetaxel (Taxotere)

Vindesine (Eldisine)

Paclitaxel (Paclitaxel, Taxol)

Vinorelbine (Navelbine)

Vinblastine (Velbe)

Targeted therapies

Alemtuzumab (MabCampath)

Lapatinib (Tykerb)

Bevacizumab (Avastin)

Nilotinib (Tasigna)

Bortezomib (Velcade)

Panitumumab (Vectibix)

Cetuximab (Erbitux)

Pazopanib (Votrient)

Erlotinib (Tarceva)

Rituximab (MabThera)

Everolimus (Afinitor)

Sorafinib (Nexavar)

Gefitinib (Iressa)

Imatinib (Glivec)

Sunitinib (Sutent)

Temsirolimus (Torisel)

Trastuzumab (Herceptin)

Cytokines

Interferon alpha (IntronA, Roferon-A, Viraferon)

Interleukin, aldesleukin (Proleukin)

Sex hormones and hormone antagonists

Abiraterone (Zytiga)

Anastrazole (Arimidex)

Bicalutamide (Casodex)

Buserilin (Suprefact)

Cyproterone acetate (Cyprostat)

Degarelix (Firmagen)

Exemestane (Aromasin)

Flutamide (Drogenil)

Fulvestrant (Faslodex)

Goserelin (Zoladex)

Letrozole (Femara)

Leuprorelin (Prostap)

Medroxyprogesterone (Farlutal, Provera)

Megestrol acetate (Megace)

Stilboestrol (Diethylstilboestrol)

Tamoxifen (Nolvadex-D)

Triptorelin (Decapeptyl, Gonapeptyl)

Appendix B: Acronyms of Some Commonly Used Cytotoxic Chemotherapy Regimens

Acronym	Drugs used	Indication(s)
ABVD	Doxorubicin (**A**driamycin), **b**leomycin, **v**inblastine, **D**acarbazine	Hodgkin lymphoma
AC	Doxorubicin (**A**driamycin), **c**yclophosphamide	Breast cancer
ACE	Doxorubicin (**A**driamycin), **c**yclophosphamide, **e**toposide	Small-cell lung

AT	Doxorubicin (**A**driamycin), docetaxel (**T**axotere)	Breast cancer
BEACOPP	**B**leomycin, **e**toposide, doxorubicin (**A**driamycin), **c**yclophosphamide, vincristine (**O**ncovin), **p**rocarbazine, **p**rednisone	Hodgkin lymphoma
BEP	**B**leomycin, **e**toposide, **c**isplatin	Testicular cancer
C-VAMP	**C**yclophosphamide, **v**incristine, doxorubicin (**A**driamycin), **m**ethyl-**p**rednisolone	Multiple myeloma
CAF	**C**yclophosphamide, doxorubicin (**A**driamycin), **F**luorouraci	Breast cancer
CarboMV	**Carbo**platin, **m**ethotrexate, **v**inblastine	Bladder cancer
CAV	**C**yclophosphamide, doxorubicin (**A**driamycin), **v**incristine	Small cell lung cancer
ChlVPP	**Chl**orambucil, **v**inblastine, **p**rocarbazine, **p**rednisolone	Hodgkin lymphoma
CHOP[a]	**C**yclophosphamide, doxorubicin (doxorubicin **h**ydrochloride), vincristine (**O**ncovin), **p**rednisolone	Non-Hodgkin lymphoma
CMF	**C**yclophosphamide, **m**ethotrexate, **f**luorouracil	Breast cancer
CYVADIC	**C**yclophosphamide, **v**incristine, doxorubicin (**A**driamycin), dacarbazine (**DTIC**)	Soft-tissue sarcoma
de Gramont	Leucovorin, bolus fluorouracil, 22 h infusion fluorouracil on days 1 and 2, every 14 days	Colorectal cancer
DHAP[a]	**D**examet**h**asone, cytarabine (cytosine **a**rabinoside), Cis**p**latin	Non-Hodgkin lymphoma
E-CMF	**E**pirubicin, **c**yclophosphamide, **m**ethotrexate, **f**luorouracil	Breast cancer
EC	**E**pirubicin, **c**yclophosphamide	Breast cancer

EC	Etoposide, cisplatin	Small cell lung cancer
ECF	Epirubicin, cisplatin, fluorouracil	Stomach, oesophageal and ovarian cancer
ECX	Epirubicin, cisplatin, capecitabine (Xeloda)	Stomach, oesophageal cancer
EEX	Epirubicin, oxaliplatin (Eloxatin), capecitabine (Xeloda)	Stomach, oesophageal cancer
ELF	Etoposide, leucovorin, fluorouracil	Stomach, oesophageal cancer
FAM	Fluorouracil, doxorubicin (Adriamycin), Mitomycin	Stomach, pancreatic cancer
FEC	Fluorouracil, epirubicin, cyclophosphamide	Breast cancer
FOLFOX	Leucovorin (folinic acid), fluorouracil, oxaliplatin	Colorectal cancer
FOLFIRI	Leucovorin (folinic acid), fluorouracil, irinotecan	Colorectal cancer
Gemcap	Gemcitabine, capecitabine	Pancreatic cancer
Gemcarbo	Gemcitabine, carboplatin	Small cell and non-small-cell lung cancer
Gemcis	Gemcitabine, cisplatin	Pancreatic and non-small-cell lung cancer
ICE[a]	Ifosfamide, carboplatin, etoposide	Small-cell lung cancer, non-Hodgkin lymphoma
MACOP-B	Methotrexate, doxorubicin (Adriamycin), cyclophosphamide, vincristine (Oncovin), prednisolone, bleomycin	Non-Hodgkin lymphoma

Mayo bolus	Fluorouracil and leucovorin daily for 5 days once every 4 weeks	Colorectal cancer
Modified de Gramont	Leucovorin, bolus fluorouracil, 46 h infusion fluorouracil on day 1, every 14 days	Colorectal cancer
MOPP	Nitrogen **m**ustard, **v**incristine (**O**ncovin), **p**rocarbazine, **p**rednisolone	Hodgkin lymphoma
M-VAC	**M**ethotrexate, **v**inblastine, doxorubicin (**A**driamycin), **C**isplatin	Bladder cancer
PCV	**P**rocarbazine, lomustine (**C**CNU), **v**incristine	Brain tumours
PMitCEBO	**P**rednisolone, **mit**oxantrone, **c**yclophosphamide, **e**toposide, **b**leomycin, vincristine (**O**ncovin)	Non-Hodgkin lymphoma
TAC	Docetaxel (**T**axotere), doxorubicin (**A**driamycin), **c**yclophosphamide	Breast cancer
VAD	**V**incristine, doxorubicin (**A**driamycin), **d**examethasone	Multiple myeloma
VAPEC-B	**V**incristine, doxorubicin (**A**driamycin), **p**rednisolone, **e**toposide, **c**yclophosphamide, **b**leomycin	Hodgkin lymphoma and non-Hodgkin lymphoma

[a]R-CHOP, R-DHAP and R-ICE are the same as these combinations with the addition of rituximab

Index

Printed by Printforce, the Netherlands